"Renowned dietitian, Georgie Fear, weaves intuitive wisdom with scientific-based evidence in her latest book. In this well written guide to healthy eating habits, Georgie spells out the process by which the readers can stop dieting and start eating healthy. Stop struggling with your diet and embrace the wisdom of a nutrition expert."

—DEVON GOLEM, PHD, RD, LD, Assistant Professor of Human Nutrition at New Mexico State University

"Georgie Fear is an incredibly bright dietician that I know and trust when it comes to nutrition. Her approach to nutrition and behavioral change in Lean Habits parallels the methods I use in my clinic, which have consistently proven successful with my patients. If you can't work one on one with an expert, this book is a great way to see exactly how it's done by the best in the field."

—DR. SPENCER NADOLSKY, board-certified family physician

"If you don't adopt the habits in this book, you're going to struggle. It's that simple."

—ARMI LEGGE, editor of *EvidenceMag.com*

"I didn't achieve lasting leanness until I quit dieting. Using Georgie's methods, I easily maintain a lower weight and body fat percentage than I thought possible when dieting. The beauty of Georgie's habits-based approach is that it's rewarding from the start. When you feel better, you do better."

—RENEE CLOE, founder of the non-dieting community HappyEaters.net.

"Georgie provides an evidence-based, thoughtful approach that allows individuals to better understand their dietary downfalls and to give their diet a makeover for life. The book addresses a topic which we all take very personally—our nutrition and our weight—and takes the guesswork out of better eating."

—MALISSA J. WOOD, MD FACC FASE FAHA, co-director MGH Heart Center Corrigan Women's Heart Health Program, co-author of *THINFLUENCE*

"Life-long nutritional success comes from acquiring healthy habits, not going 'on' and 'off' the latest fad diet du jour. *Lean Habits* offers a smart list of healthy habits you can acquire for a lifetime of lean and optimal eating."

—SHARON PALMER, RDN, author of *Plant-Powered for Life*

LEAN
HABITS
FOR LIFELONG
WEIGHT LOSS

PAGE STREET
PUBLISHING CO.

First published in 2015 by
Page Street Publishing Co.
27 Congress Street, Suite 103
Salem, MA 01970
www.pagestreetpublishing.com

Distributed by Macmillan; sales in Canada by The Canadian Manda Group; distribution in Canada by The Jaguar Book Group.

18   17   16   15   1   2   3   4   5

ISBN-13: 978-1-62414-112-6
ISBN-10: 1-62414-112-9

Library of Congress Control Number: 2014946087

Cover and book design by Page Street Publishing Co.
Cover photography by Brian T. Wolf

Printed and bound in the United States

Page Street is proud to be a member of 1% for the Planet. Members donate one percent of their sales to one or more of the over 1,500 environmental and sustainability charities across the globe that participate in this program.

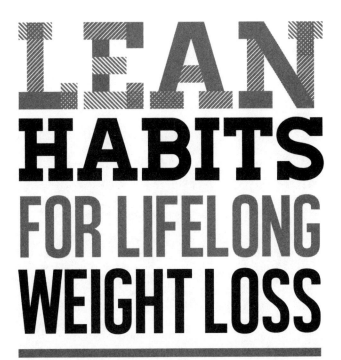

LEAN HABITS FOR LIFELONG WEIGHT LOSS

MASTERING 4 CORE EATING BEHAVIORS TO STAY SLIM FOREVER

GEORGIE FEAR

REGISTERED DIETITIAN, NUTRITION EXPERT AND CO-AUTHOR OF *RACING WEIGHT COOKBOOK*

PAGE STREET
PUBLISHING CO.

CONTENTS

CORE HABITS

SUPPORTING HABITS

FOREWORD

I was training for the Olympics in cross-country skiing. In my twice-daily workouts, I imagined my dream coming true: I would race for Canada in my third Olympics in Sochi, Russia.

The only things that could stop me were my mental and physical health problems. For two years, I'd had a very difficult relationship with food. I needed to find the balance between feelings and food in order to get my mind and body working together.

Enter nutrition coach extraordinaire Georgie Fear.

Georgie, with her inspiring physique and a thousand-watt smile, transformed my life, health and performance. My health today is a testament to the lasting change her work can bring, and the exciting fact that *anyone* can do it. Diets didn't work; *Lean Habits* did.

Excellent fueling is essential for high-performance sport. The word "diet," with its connotation of futility, was never used on the ski team. However, measuring out 12 almonds as my fat allocation for a certain meal, or frying up a cup of egg whites and vegetables for breakfast certainly brings the word "diet" to mind. Some worked, some didn't.

The real problems came when, a couple years before the 2014 Olympics, a traumatic breakup with my then-boyfriend swept me up in a powerful current of negative emotion. For a year, I suffered bouts of bulimia that eventually destroyed my body's ability to perform as a ski racer.

Thank goodness for Georgie Fear.

The first thing I noticed was the pure, flawless logic of Georgie's advice. If my eating behaviors were in response to emotion, then attempting to solve them this way was akin to attempting to start my car engine by honking the horn: useless at best. In the case of my calamitous personal life, my responses made a bad situation worse.

With patience and compassion, Georgie guided me with easy-to-understand psychology and physiology as well as great anecdotes from her decades of coaching experience. She offered great support and frequent course corrections through setbacks, and my life was transformed.

The pages of this book contain everything you need to transform your life. The habits make so much sense and work so well, I know you can make lasting changes to your life. Diets don't work; *Lean Habits* does.

It's been a year since the end of my professional ski racing career, and the strength of the habits I cultivated now feel as undeniable as gravity. I'm as happy with my lean habits as I am with the way my smallest jeans fit.

As for my dream? In February 2014 I skied across the snow of the Olympic cross-country stadium in Sochi, Russia, and achieved my dream. My mind and body were completely in sync. *Lean Habits* helped me live my dream and they'll help you with yours too.

All the best with your new habits,
Chandra

ABOUT THIS BOOK

Lean Habits is a proven, evidence-based system for losing fat, one habit at a time. As opposed to a "diet," which typically provides an overwhelming, uncomfortable and temporary weight-loss strategy, this habit-based weight-loss system utilizes research into what actually works to help achieve lifelong leanness. The Lean Habits system presented in this book capitalizes on the latest nutrition research, while integrating critical components of change psychology, positive psychology and the neurological basis of habit. One habit at a time, this book will coach you through adopting various nutritional and lifestyle habits. The Lean Habits system has already been proven tremendously successful by hundreds of clients I have worked with over the years, normal, everyday people just like you. The book you're holding right now will help *you* achieve the same life-changing results, without having to hire a professional weight-loss coach.

In each chapter, we'll focus on one Lean Habit, a behavior that's been proven to help people get and stay lean. I'll walk you through the practical steps involved in adopting the habit (What to Do) and show you how to keep track of your practice. Then I'll explain the rationale behind each one (Why It's Worth It), followed by a discussion on the mechanisms at work (How It Works). Potential challenges you may encounter will be discussed, as well as ways you can scale the habit upward or downward to tailor it to the perfect level of challenge for you. The Lean Habits system will develop more than just your eating skills; you'll hone mental strategies—for example, how to handle family dynamics at holiday dinners and manage emotional ups and downs without turning to food.

One of the most important—and awesome—concepts to grasp is that you do not have to suffer through calorie counting, social isolation, cumbersome calculations or deprivation to lose fat. Attaining and maintaining a lean, healthy body can be as effortless and automatic as brushing your teeth once the right habits have been formed, and this book will take you through the daily practice and motivation you need to form those habits. Instead of trying to do it all at once, you'll find that having an expert coach prioritize a single thing to do at a time makes the potentially overwhelming journey of changing many habits doable. With Lean Habits, your dieting days are over.

I'm a professional weight-loss coach. I'm going to still be part of the weight loss marketplace next year, and the one after that. My goal is that you, however, *aren't*.

INTRODUCTION

FAT LOSS: WHAT'S THE PROBLEM?

How is it that the U.S. diet industry makes $20 billion annually while more than one in three adults (35 percent) remains obese? Is it that people just don't care? Not likely. According to consumer market research, 20 percent of people are on a diet at any given time, and the typical dieter makes four to five attempts each year to lose weight. That means *four to five times a year* they failed to achieve their goal but did not give up. That says to me that people really do care. They care enough to try again about every two months, in many cases for years on end. This is interesting, considering that most industries or businesses that fail to produce results for a majority of their customers would be out of business rapidly. Yet not the weight-loss industry—people keep coming back, with hope that this next diet will be the one.

You probably know dozens of people who have lost weight temporarily, but regained it. You may in fact be one of them. This is typical actually. Fad diets that are meant to be done for a short period of time are logically only good for short-term results. So the *7-Day Detox Miracle* likely doesn't surprise or disappoint many consumers by not helping them achieve permanent control over their weight. It's likely that people seeking quick fixes are thinking short term anyway—i.e., looking good on a specific day, such as for a reunion or wedding.

If we set aside short-term fixes, like weeklong liquid fasts and extreme 30-day regimens, and look at methods meant to be followed for a longer period of time, would the results be more promising? Unfortunately, looking only at dieters who intend to make a lifestyle change shows that many people simply don't stay on a diet long enough to see the initial results. Polls indicate that the average woman will last just under three weeks each time she tries to diet, most of those efforts being do-it-yourself stints.

Assuming that a person is wise enough to avoid temporary quick-fix products and decides to work with a registered dietitian or enroll in a well-designed weight-loss program through a research university to help her stick with her behavioral change beyond the initial weeks, things *should* work out for her, right? Sadly, these methods also produce disappointing long-term results.

After analyzing 31 weight-loss studies, researchers at UCLA concluded that people typically lose 5 to 10 percent of their initial body weight in the first six months of a diet. However, anywhere from 30 to 60 percent of them regain every single ounce of it. In one report, 83 percent of people gained back more weight than they had lost when followed for four years. And 50 percent of the people weighed eleven pounds or more *above their starting weight* four years after going on a weight-loss diet.

Does this pattern of weight loss and regain sound familiar? If so, you know it's no laughing matter. When it's your life, your self-esteem and your health on the line, failing to lose weight and keep it off is more than frustrating, it's maddening—even devastating.

The cutting edge of weight-management research today is looking *beyond diets*, because it's clear that diets do not provide a lasting solution to a person's weight problem. It is increasingly apparent to experts that adherence is king; therefore, behavioral science and psychology will play a critical part in the next horizons of obesity management. After all, the most consistent finding of weight-loss trials is that adherence (the length of time and consistency with which you do the desired behavior) is the largest predictor of weight loss, not the specific foods you consume or nutrient ratio.

Why is lasting change so elusive when following a diet? Because sticking to a diet, is stressful. Here's how:

1. Most diets make us too physically uncomfortable to be sustainable. Most diets create a large calorie deficit in order to achieve rapid weight loss. Drastically reducing calories and keeping them low can cause the dieter to experience low energy, fatigue, constant hunger, mental fog, hair loss, decreased athletic performance, poor sleep and feelings of coldness all the time. No one will do anything forever that feels significantly unpleasant. Like a physical discomfort, mental or emotional distress can start off small but increase over time to becoming unbearable if unaddressed. It's like having a rock in your shoe to be on a diet. You handle it for a while, but eventually you want to fling it away.

2. Most diets involve a lot of change all at once, which makes us too mentally uncomfortable to sustain them. Sticking to a set meal plan or set of rules feels foreign and artificial. We miss comforting, familiar patterns of "our" way of eating: the breakfast we're used to having, our favorite family recipes and our holiday traditions.

3. Most diets decrease our quality of life more than we're willing to put up with forever. Not only do we miss out on our favorite foods when dieting, but sticking to a rigid restrictive plan often means being left out of fun and meaningful experiences like the impromptu frozen yogurt date or sampling a treat your child baked just for you. Lack of dietary variety can induce low mood, irritability, boredom and, especially if you're a "foodie," can mean loss of a pleasurable hobby in cooking. We also get tired of working so hard to count points and tally calories; we long to use that willpower for other areas of life.

Despite all of this, people still come to me wanting me to make a meal plan for them. Some still want to be put on a diet (meaning a temporary regimen to get pounds off, after which they will stop doing it). Many people imply or say outright that they would love for me to give them a calorie total to shoot for, tell them which foods to banish from their homes and which can stay, or crack down on them and slap the doughnut out of their hand so they can finally stop eating sugar.

As a logical argument, the idea that dieting is the only way to lose weight is so flawed that it's almost laughable—in no small part because dieting works so rarely, and most of us have personal experience to confirm that. We don't even need to take someone else's word. Why then would bright, capable, successful people who have been failed by every diet they've ever tried want more of the same? It's because society has told all of us over and over again that this is the only road to a lean body.

If you want to lose weight, it's normal to assume that rules and rigid restrictions are necessary because alternatives are seldom provided or even mentioned. The brainwashing message pumped out in unison by advertising firms, magazine articles and even personal trainers is that you either eat whatever and stay fat, or diet and get thin. This dichotomy leaves little consolation or explanation for the millions of people who *are dieting* and not losing any weight. It leaves dieters to come up with their own conclusions as to why their hard work hasn't yielded the promised results. If "diets work" is what we hear a dozen times a day, but you've been dieting and it's *not working*, what are you to believe? Individuals typically infer that they must have done something wrong and not dieted correctly, or that another diet would be substantially different and they must have gotten the wrong set of rigid rules this time. Instead of Paleo, they try Weight Watchers, or South Beach, or the Dukan Diet, or intermittent fasting.

There isn't a concise, four-letter word that encompasses the process I promote, the alternative to *diet*. The anti-diet concept that I have spent years working to understand, study and communicate is the idea of changing yourself as an eater. Following a meal plan or eating prepackaged diet food for a few weeks is a lot less threatening than the idea of shaping different attitudes and behaviors. Changing yourself sounds, for lack of a better term, really freakin' hard. But there is a gleam in my eye, a spark of hope that I happily share with you: it's not that bad. In fact, it's pretty awesome. When you have a supportive guide, a clear roadmap to follow and can go at your own pace, changing yourself ends up being a natural, rewarding and effective strategy—three things that I have not heard said about dieting.

My clients' success with lasting weight loss comes from combining the latest in nutritional science, change psychology and behavior change into a system that's practical, simple and makes cementing permanent behaviors almost effortless. **Above all, the Lean Habits system avoids the things that make following a diet so highly stressful: physical discomfort, sweeping sudden changes to your lifestyle and psychological burden are all kept as low as possible.**

WHY HABITS?

Using the Lean Habits, you'll find it's possible to do things differently than you have before, in a way that minimizes the above three issues. We'll be taking change one habit at a time. Unlike attempting to completely overhaul your lifestyle, focusing on one detail at a time dramatically increases your chances of success. It enables you to concentrate your efforts on truly mastering a skill, repeating it enough that it becomes easy, intuitive and nearly effortless. This minimizes the physical and mental discomfort of losing weight. Incremental change and flexible behavior goals are far less stress-inducing.

A lower stress burden not only makes this system more pleasant, but also more effective. Research shows that individuals who seek to lose weight by adopting rigid rules or following a diet are more prone to binge eating and weight gain than individuals who aren't trying to restrict their intake. Stress increases appetite and fat storage, and weakens willpower and tenacity in the face of a challenge. In other words, trying to diet in an inflexible manner may be the worst thing you could do for your waistline.

Think about how automatically you brush your teeth each morning; even half-asleep, you can get that done. What if *all* the things you needed to do to lose weight were equally automatic? They wouldn't require willpower, restraint or tons of obsessive thinking. You wouldn't stress over whether you could do them each day, worry about how long you could keep this up or panic when a vacation came up. Like brushing your teeth, you'd just do them.

I've been doing exactly that, changing one habit at a time, with hundreds of people and the results are pretty astounding.

CONCEPTUAL FRAMEWORK

The Lean Habits system was built with one primary endpoint in mind: to make fat loss as effortless and as pleasant as possible. It's important to me to not just get people lean, but to help them enjoy their lives more, which meant methods that required lots of suffering were out. I wouldn't sleep well at night if I knew my clients were sacrificing life quality to put my advice into place. I want to make people's lives better, not worse.

The science that went into the development of the Lean Habits system focuses on maximizing appetite satisfaction and enhancing experiential satisfaction. In my career as a professional nutrition counselor, I have talked with thousands of people about their eating behaviors. These two themes arise again and again, in different forms—they are virtually omnipresent in conversations about why people struggle with losing weight. If you've struggled with your weight, chances are that you've experienced both types of challenge. Weight-loss methods generally fail because they leave us too physically hungry and/or we're missing some experience that food and eating used to give us.

EXPERIENTIAL SATISFACTION

I love food. Food is so much more to me than the physical nutrients it contains. Enjoying my favorite foods brings me great amounts of pleasure. I love to cook food and share food, to smell it, admire it, enjoy it on sunny picnics and savor it by candlelight. Preparing a delicious meal for myself is an act of self-care and an affirmation of my values. I also enjoy the spontaneity of my food life, to be able to accept an impromptu lunch invite or try a new restaurant with a pal and not stress over it.

I hope you love food too, and that you don't want to give up the good ways in which it adds to creating pleasurable life experiences. It's okay to love food! Joy is not fattening; in fact, the opposite is true. Having fulfilling, enjoyable experiences with food is part of a happy life and favors getting lean. As you work through the Lean Habits in this book you'll find that a recurring theme is enjoying your food more, not less.

The impact of food on our lives isn't always positive, however. Keeping experiential satisfaction high also means moving away from behaviors and thought patterns by which food *detracts* from your happiness. I went through more than a decade of life stressing over what and how much to eat because I worried that everything would make me fat. Judging myself as "good" or "bad" depending on how much I ate that day kept my happiness and self-esteem low and as fragile as glass. If food is a source of stress and guilt, or it becomes the currency by which we gauge our self-worth, it can diminish how happy we are on the whole. You may have felt or be currently experiencing ways that food and eating behaviors can cause you worry, take up excess mental focus and energy, distract you from things that *really* matter or serve as a stand-in and prevent you from learning more effective emotional coping skills. Not everyone who wants to lose weight is affected by these factors, but if you are, rest assured that the Lean Habits you're about to learn include guidance on leaving those behind too.

APPETITE SATISFACTION

Understanding how your body regulates food intake is incredibly helpful in designing meals for weight loss. If you know how your body's basic appetite-regulating circuitry operates, you can eat strategically for maximum hunger satisfaction per calorie.

First of all, understand that your brain is in charge of turning up and turning down your drive to ingest calories, as well as your energy expenditure. The hypothalamus, a central region within your brain, governs hunger and satiety signals (in addition to a host of other body systems). It's no simple task, and much more complicated than reading a fuel gauge in a car that runs from "Empty" on one side to "Full" on the other.

To give your brain the information it needs to govern your appetite and energy balance, your stomach and digestive organs are constantly sending information to the hypothalamus about how much food you've eaten, how much energy that food contains and what specific nutrients you've ingested. Between meals, they send signals that fat is being broken down and stored carbohydrate is being released. Furthermore, the hypothalamus integrates signals from the rest your body about how much stored body fat you have, how plentiful your carbohydrate stores are and what your energy-output needs are. To summarize, the appetite and satiety centers integrate complex information into the sensations we perceive as hunger and satiety. You don't reach for food because of what your stomach says, but because of what your brain perceives.

WARNING: SCIENCE AHEAD

If you're interested in understanding the biological mechanisms behind why these Lean Habits work so well at controlling appetite, they're coming up next. However, it's totally optional and if science-lingo turns you off, skip ahead to the next section, "What Does It All Mean?" (page 26). There won't be a test, and it won't hold up your success with this system.

HUNGER AND SATIETY: IT'S ALL IN YOUR HEAD

The hypothalamus contains specific neurons that make a neurotransmitter known as NPY (neuropeptide Y). This protein stimulates hunger and food intake. NPY is one of the main regulators of appetite and food intake, but other factors, including ghrelin, agouti-related protein (AgRP), orexin and melanin-concentrating hormone (MCH), contribute to the feeling of being hungry. In simple terms, think of NPY neurons as cells in your brain that make you feel hungry. When they are activated, you start hankering for a sandwich.

Other neurons in the hypothalamus—known as POMC neurons—perform the opposite function by producing a substance known as alpha melanocyte stimulating hormone (alphaMSH), a neurotransmitter that leads to satiety and suppression of appetite. When POMC neurons are activated, they suppress your appetite and give you the sensation that maybe you don't feel like that sandwich after all.

There are other signaling molecules that contribute to sensations of fullness, including corticotropin-releasing hormone (CRH) and cocaine- and amphetamine-related transcript (CART). NPY neurons and POMC neurons interact with and oppose each other, so signals from the body which activate one type of neuron typically inhibit the other "team" at the same time. For example, the appetite-suppressing hormone leptin decreases food intake by activating POMC neurons (which signal satiety) and inhibiting NPY (hunger-producing) neurons. In contrast, the appetite-stimulating hormone ghrelin inhibits POMC neurons and activates NPY neurons, which triggers you to start seeking food.

HOW YOUR GUT SIGNALS GET TO YOUR BRAIN

Feeling satisfied after a meal is more involved than simply filling up your stomach with enough volume of food. How does your brain even know what's in your stomach, anyway? After all, your brain sits a few feet higher up, in your skull, while your stomach is in your abdomen. I'll first explain how your belly "talks" to your brain. Then I'll sum up how this information is leveraged into specific Lean Habits that maximally satisfy your appetite.

The brain's hunger and satiety center gathers information from three sources:
- Direct nerve connections
- Circulating nutrients in the bloodstream
- Hormone levels in the bloodstream

DIRECT NERVE CONNECTIONS

Stretch receptors in the gastrointestinal tract do exactly what it sounds like: they pick up on the stretching of the stomach and intestinal walls and relay information to the brain about the volume of food eaten. This signal is relayed to the brain relatively rapidly via the vagus nerve, a direct nerve connection from the digestive organs to the brain (like a direct hotline).

The other two forms of gut–brain communication are slightly slower, since it takes some time for nutrients and hormones to accumulate in the bloodstream. As you can imagine, one dietary strategy to elicit this type of satiety signal in full force is eating high-volume or heavy foods like salads and vegetable soup, which place more tension on the walls of the stomach. However, if you've ever eaten mountains of lettuce in pursuit of fullness you know that you can get that "full" feeling, even see your belly distended, but while hunger is dampened you still lack a fully developed, satisfied feeling. Clearly, there is something more to feeling truly satisfied beyond filling up the stomach.

CIRCULATING NUTRIENTS

The brain has delicate sensing mechanisms to detect concentrations of glucose and fatty acids in the bloodstream, as well as certain amino acids such as leucine. There is evidence that increased concentration of circulating glucose increases the firing of appetite-suppressing POMC neurons, while reducing the rate of firing among hunger-stimulating NPY neurons. Rising concentrations of leucine appear to have a similar effect. This nutrient sensing system helps control energy intake by decreasing hunger and appetite after a meal, when circulating nutrients are at their highest. As your food starts to break down and glucose and amino acids are released into the blood, these start telling the brain that you haven't just stretched out your stomach with fizzy water or lettuce, but provided adequate calories and nutrients. This starts to turn off your appetite and trigger feelings of being satisfied.

HORMONES

Cells along the gastrointestinal tract produce a wide variety of hormones, or chemical messengers, that circulate in the bloodstream in response to food intake. The signal can reach the brain in one of two ways: hormones can bind to receptors on nerves in the gut that transmit electrical impulses to the brain, or the hormones can circulate to the brain via the bloodstream and bind to receptors there. The following are some of the hormones involved in appetite regulation.

GLP-1 (glucagon-like peptide 1): This protein is secreted from intestinal L cells in response to nutrients entering the intestines. Carbohydrates, protein and fat all elicit GLP-1 production. GLP-1 reduces hunger and food intake by binding to a receptor in the hypothalamus. It also helps trigger insulin release. Insulin and GLP-1 both suppress ghrelin, a hormone that triggers sensations of hunger. Fat has been shown to stimulate GLP-1 more than a calorically equivalent amount of carbohydrate.

GIP (glucose-dependent insulinotropic polypeptide): Produced by K cells in the first part of the small intestine, GIP secretion is regulated mostly by the carbohydrate concentration inside the intestine. It is not known for certain whether GIP directly suppresses appetite in the central nervous system or if it boosts satiety indirectly through enhancing the insulin response.

Oxyntomodulin and peptide tyrosine tyrosine (PYY): Secreted from L cells in the distal intestine, both of these hormones contribute to satisfaction and also slow the rate of stomach emptying, contributing to a longer-lasting feeling of fullness and less dramatic rise in blood glucose. High-protein meals stimulate greater PYY release than high-carbohydrate or high-fat meals. Fat also has been shown to cause greater circulating increases in PYY than carbohydrates. PYY has been shown to stimulate the vagus nerve while oxyntomodulin acts directly on the hypothalamic neurons using the same receptors as GLP-1.

Cholecystokinin (CCK): Released by I cells in response to free fatty acids and amino acids appearing in the small intestine, CCK decreases appetite in two ways—by binding to receptors in the brain and by stimulating activity of the vagus nerve. Consuming protein-rich foods with meals stimulates CCK most effectively.

Leptin: This hormone is secreted from fat tissue as well as the stomach and other digestive organs. Levels of circulating leptin correlate with levels of body fat. Leptin acts to decrease energy intake and promote weight loss by stimulating release of alphaMSH and inhibiting NPY production in the hypothalamus. Leptin also suppresses orexin (another appetite-stimulating neurotransmitter) and extinguishes the food-reward response in the brain, essentially helping you put the fork down. Interestingly, certain individuals show an increase in circulating leptin levels during a stressful event, while others have a reduced response, a phenomenon which may explain why some people "stress-eat" high-fat, high-sugar foods more than others. Leptin levels also typically peak at night (presumably an adaptation to allow sleep without being woken by hunger). Individuals who have compulsive night-eating syndrome have been shown to have a lesser degree of leptin increase at night, which may partially explain the development of the disorder. Keeping your body sensitive to leptin helps it do its job, curbing your appetite when you take in calorie excess and stimulating physical activity to burn it off. Adequate sleep, as you'll see, is a key habit in maintaining leptin sensitivity.

Secretin: Produced by S cells in the intestine, secretin has been shown to alter hypothalamic activity and reduce food intake by increasing impulses along the vagus nerve, activating POMC neurons. The products of fat and protein digestion stimulate its release, as well as the drop in pH from stomach acid.

Ghrelin: Also known as the hunger hormone, ghrelin is unlike all the previously mentioned chemical messengers in that it stimulates appetite and increases food intake. Levels of ghrelin peak before a meal and fall with food intake.

WHAT DOES IT ALL MEAN?

The complicated system we just reviewed actually boils down to just a small number of key dietary factors. To maximize your physical satisfaction for every calorie, you need to:

1. Build meals with enough weight and volume
2. Get enough protein
3. Consume the right amount of fat
4. Eat adequate carbohydrates
5. Maintain your leptin sensitivity
6. Avoid blood sugar instability (and the excess hunger it causes)

The Lean Habits system teaches you, one habit at a time, exactly how to eat to achieve all those endpoints.

WHERE WE'LL START: AT THE BEGINNING

One of the most common mistakes people make in a weight-loss or habit-change program is prioritizing ineffectively. Trying to fine-tune the details before the big, important habits are in place is a surefire way to waste effort and an inefficient road to progress at best. Starting in the right place and progressing logically is highly influential on whether your efforts will be effective and rewarding, or downright frustrating.

I hear every day from individuals who are struggling to master details of their diet when they've never addressed the big, glaring holes in their nutrition strategy. In *Lean Habits*, we'll start with the foundational habits that are most important to get in place from the outset. The first section will assist you with identifying, getting comfortable with and utilizing your body's internal signals to help you lose weight. From there, we'll move into more detail about how you can easily achieve a calorie deficit (without counting calories) by maximizing the appetite satisfaction you get from each calorie by smart food choices. We'll also explore how flexibility and treats fit in, and what lifestyle factors keep appetite signals appropriately calibrated.

The Lean Habits are delivered in a specific order to maximize your results and eliminate spinning your wheels as much as possible. I encourage you to not skip habits or rush to the next habit because you don't particularly like one. It's helpful to keep in mind that the habits that challenge you the most also are often the most productive behavior changes in unlocking your results. And while it's best to not eliminate or skip habits, I strongly encourage you to customize the level of challenge at each step by scaling the change.

SCALING A HABIT

Habits in this book should not be interpreted as hard-and-fast rules that immediately take effect when you turn the page. If a habit is too hard, and your confidence isn't high enough that it sounds like something you can do, you'll have a much better chance at success by scaling down the challenge into something you are confident you can do. I'll give you an example: one Lean Habit discusses minimizing liquid calories. If you feel ready to grab the bull by the horns and switch to drinking nothing but water, that's great. But if you're not sure that you can or want to do that in one step, I encourage you to scale the habit. It may be more realistic to think about cutting the amount of juice you drink in half, or focus on switching from sweetened tea to unsweetened tea first, and tackling your juice calories separately. It's better to take a small step you are confident in than attempt a big leap you have little faith in landing.

Consider what level of difficulty or amount of change feels doable for you, and scale habits as needed to provide a level of challenge that you are confident you can consistently practice. One thing I routinely ask my clients is, "On a scale of zero to 10 (zero being not confident at all, and 10 being positive you can nail this), how confident are you that you can practice this habit almost every day, if not every day, for the next two weeks?" If they answer anything below a 9, we have work to do, either by shrinking the change to make the habit easier or by removing a barrier.

If someone states that they are 8-out-of-10 confident they can get vegetables into their lunches each day, then continuing the conversation might reveal that one of their barriers is that they eat from the office cafeteria, which has only limp, overcooked vegetables. However, we can work around that barrier by adding baby carrots and radishes to their weekly shopping list and planning to make five individual bags of veggies Sunday night to grab each morning to bring to work. With a concrete plan, the client's confidence often rises to 9 or 10. I recommend you do the same as you work through this book, playing the role of your own coach. Assess your confidence as you prepare to tackle each new habit, and if you feel less than 9-out-of-10 confident, shrink the change or think about what barriers you can remove or work around.

ACCOUNTABILITY AND HABIT TRACKING

Once you've got your first Lean Habit to work on, you'll need some way to keep yourself accountable. I recommend starting an Excel spreadsheet or using a paper notebook. Across the top of the page, write the dates for the next 14 days. On the left, you'll write your habit. Each day, all you have to do is mark down an *x* to indicate you practiced your habit. As you progress and add a second habit, you can write it underneath the first.

HABIT	1	2	3	4	5	6	7	8	9	10	11	12	13	14
Habit 1	x	x	x		x	x								
Habit 2	x		x	x	x	x								
Habit 3	x	x	x	x	x	x								

Tracking habits works. Saying "I'll just do it in my head" or "I'll just try and cut back" rarely works, if ever. When you're practicing a new behavior, black-and-white evidence goes a long way. You'll know whether you're actually changing your habits or squandering your efforts just trying but not actually making any changes.

Trying to change your habits doesn't take weight off. You have to actually practice your habits, so make sure you write them down somewhere to keep track.

Another reason to keep an accurate record of your habit practice as you go is that it's absolutely essential for maintaining your early habits after you've progressed to adding others. If you forget what you did earlier, you might only remember the most recent habit. Then, if you start to slip back to your old ways on a previously covered habit, you might end up confused and unsure what changed that halted your progress. Keeping a good record will make it easy to see exactly what combination of behaviors works for you, so you can troubleshoot down the road.

Handy tip: some smartphone apps can help you keep track of your habits, so consider using your phone if it's always by your side. Check out HabitList.com for one app that can help you record your progress.

Last, recording each x in your habit tracker functions as a small reward. There is a positive psychological effect of seeing our diligent efforts add up. Each time you practice your habit, give yourself a pat on the back, a little "heck yeah, go me!" and let yourself feel a little jazzed about it. Positive reinforcement hastens the formation of habit. So go ahead, have a little mental parade in your honor each and every time you nail your habit. It's okay, no one will know.

PRACTICE, NOT PERFECTION

If you slip up a little and have a mixture of success and failure in a given week, that's normal! Be nice to yourself. You don't have to nail every habit 100 percent of the time to be getting better at it, and given enough time, you're bound to have a day of missing your habit sooner or later. Instead of expecting yourself to ace every habit from day one, give yourself time to practice and improve your skill with each habit, and it will get easier. If you already knew how to do it, you wouldn't be practicing.

If you are trying to practice a certain behavior each time you eat, then you have several *opportunities* a day to practice. I had the opportunity to go to several lectures a day when I was an undergraduate student, and while I went to most of them, occasionally I let one slip by for some extra sleep. And what happened? I emerged with a great education, an excellent grade-point average and went to graduate school at a top Ivy League university. It's okay if you don't have a perfect record.

You might also visualize practicing your habits like practicing your tennis backhand with a tennis ball machine. The machine will keep serving you balls, and one or two are bound to whizz by you in the course of your practice. It doesn't mean you aren't getting any better or that practice session was a waste! Just keep at it. One of the great things about working on our nutrition habits is that we get to practice every single day because we eat every single day. I'm glad I'm not a python who eats once every three months; even if I don't eat in line with my intentions at one meal, I get a chance in just a number of hours to nail it with a do-over.

KEEP SLIPUPS IN PERSPECTIVE

Changing behaviors and habits is *hard*, even more so when the habits surround something as emotional and personal as food and our body weight. Many people think they will be able to just stop all of their old behaviors cold turkey once they commit to new ones. While this is an enthusiastic and positive outlook, it's not the most realistic way to expect your journey to go, especially if you've been battling maladaptive food behaviors your entire life! Some habits you might pick up and soar with from day one, but on the whole that's pretty unlikely. **Your experience with most habits will involve some missteps. That's perfectly okay. It's the only way, in fact, to learn that you won't fall apart when you fall short of your intention.** You're not made of glass; you won't shatter. You'll get back up and keep practicing and be fine. (In fact, if one my clients gets upset at wrecking their perfect streak, I congratulate them on finally bringing real life into the journey: "Awesome, now you can stop trying to be perfect! This just got real, now you can learn your own resilience.")

IDEALIZED PROGRESS MAY LOOK LIKE THIS IN YOUR MIND

Before:

Screw up ➜ feel bad about my screwup so I screw up more ➜ feel even worse about myself ➜ keep screwing up ➜ divine intervention or serious wake-up call ➜ get back on track days or weeks after initial slip.

After:

No screwup, ever.

Well, that *would* be nice. It's not how actual humans change, though. In real life, improvement from that "before" situation looks more like this:

Stage 1: Screw up ➜ feel bad about my screwup so I screw up more ➜ feel even worse about myself ➜ remember I don't have to keep doing this ➜ get back on track without waiting for divine intervention or rock bottom (maybe the next day).

Stage 2: Screw up ➜ feel bad about my screwup so I screw up more ➜ see where this is going ➜ remember I don't have to keep doing this ➜ get back on track (possibly the same day).

Stage 3: Screw up ➜ start to feel bad but realize it was just a mistake ➜ realize I can stop now without making my situation worse ➜ get back on track right away.

Stage 4: Start to screw up ➜ realize (perhaps halfway through the piece of cheesecake I didn't even want but am eating anyway) that I don't have to keep doing this ➜ abort screwup and get back on track.

Stage 5: Consider screwup ➜ remember that never works ➜ decide otherwise.

As you can see, there are many steps separating a cyclical trap of mistakes and guilt and a fictional ideal of rarely making a mistake because you know better. Even after a person gets to that stage 5 experience the first time, they still typically dabble in stage 4 for a bit (almost like we just need a bit more evidence that a certain choice doesn't work out so well). It's okay to always be a work in progress. I assure you, it does get easier, and your missteps get fewer and further between as you observe your outcomes, forgive yourself and keep perspective.

Here's a big secret: you don't have to be 100 percent perfect at these habits. *Ever.* Working up to 90 percent or greater consistency on the Lean Habits is highly correlated with weight-loss success, but missing one mark here and there is fabulously non-disastrous. Just get back to it the next day, and luckily, there's always another opportunity to practice. Don't put pressure on yourself; it's just *practice.* These habits work to get you lean and keep you lean if you practice them *most* of the time. But they aren't hard-and-fast rules with zero exceptions.

FOR HOW LONG DO I PRACTICE EACH LEAN HABIT?

Give yourself a minimum of 14 days to practice each habit before adding the next one. You can certainly take more time than that, but the goal is to not just "get a grip" on each behavior before moving on, but to do it enough that it becomes *incredibly easy*, almost automatic. That often means reining in your enthusiasm to add the next habit as soon as you have a basic proficiency of the current one. Give yourself time and, for your own good, be patient enough.

Phase 1: The habit will feel difficult and take deliberate effort.

Phase 2: The habit will feel easy, but still deliberate. This is a tempting time to add the next habit, but stick it out.

Phase 3: The habit becomes automatic, and happens without you thinking about it. Now, it's a much better time to add the next habit.

When your current habit feels truly automatic and habitual without thinking about it, then it's time to move to the next one. Feel free to take more than two weeks with particularly challenging habits, or to repeat an old habit if you find you need a refresher. There is no rush. My clients often return to focus on foundational habits if they find their weight loss has stalled; with a brushup on the basics, they are able to get their weight loss moving once again.

You'll know you are progressing too quickly if any of your daily behaviors as recorded on your tracker are slipping and being successfully completed less than 80 percent of the time. If that happens, don't add any more habits until you're able to be more consistent with the ones you are already tracking. And if you find you went a bit fast out of the gate (whoops, maybe I added too much too fast!), just dial back and reduce the number of habits to allow more time to focus on adopting each one singly.

HOW MUCH WEIGHT CAN I EXPECT TO LOSE, AND HOW FAST?

Consistently doing all of the Lean Habits has been proven with thousands of clients to result in a steady weight loss of one-half to one pound a week, but your results may be faster or more gradual. Your body may begin changing shape after the very first habit, or it may take the accumulated change of several habits before your behaviors are consistently producing enough of a calorie deficit to start seeing pounds drop.

Why does this vary so much person to person? The behaviors that produced the body you currently have are not the same as everyone else who wants to lose weight. You may only have one or two "problem" habits, and changing those one or two keystones yields weight loss. If you have a multitude of bad habits that are all contributing to excess weight, it means you need to be a bit patient as we amend them one by one. Once you've reached a critical mass of behavior change, your body *will change*.

Instead of focusing on your weight and whether it is changing or not, I recommend focusing on the behaviors you are working on and doing them as consistently as possible. If you don't want to weigh yourself and can observe changes in your body in the mirror and your clothes, that will work. If you do want to monitor your weight, I strongly recommend weighing yourself no more than once a week. Weighing yourself every single day may feel like it helps "keep you on track," but it actually makes it harder for you to make the consistent behavior changes that you need to lose weight, in addition to placing an undue emotional burden on you that is unhelpful and unnecessary. If you currently get on the scale every day and are wincing at the idea of starting a day without that seemingly critical piece of information, consider facing that fear and using it as an indicator of readiness to change. If you've struggled unsuccessfully to lose weight, and you've stepped on the scale every day for years, the obsession doesn't appear to be helping you learn, does it? Daily weigh-ins may have ruined a lot of mornings for you that would otherwise have been more enjoyable. The intrusion of a numerical assessment each day also gets in the way of embarking on your day with a self-concept based on who you are and the behaviors you desire. You don't need the number every day; what you need is to know what you want to do today. If you want to know "how am I doing?" just look at your habit tracker and see if you are practicing the behaviors as consistently as possible.

There are two ways that weighing yourself too often can impede your progress.

If you have not lost weight or see that your weight has gone up, it's easy to feel negative, wonder if you can't do this or question if the habits are working. That makes it harder to do your habit today. These habits do work to get people leaner, but weight loss does not happen every single day in a linear fashion. Everyone's weight varies several pounds from day to day; even those who are losing weight successfully have days and weeks where their weight is higher than it was at the last measurement.

If your weight is down, it's easy to think "I'm doing well, I've been good, I can cheat today and not do my habit." Obviously, this overconfidence leading to self-sabotage halts weight loss from continuing. If it's working, that's great, but you need to keep doing the Lean Habits for it to keep working!

Measure your weight once a week. If you like, you can record circumference measurements as well, using a flexible tape measure to determine the girth of your hips, thighs and midsection. But if you want the lowest burden of data to collect, just hop on the scale once a week, jot it down and put it out of your mind. What you really need to focus on is changing behaviors.

So it's about time for us to talk about exactly that, the first Lean Habit.

LEAN HABIT 1:

EAT 3 OR 4 MEALS PER DAY WITHOUT SNACKING

WHAT TO DO

Factor in adjustments to your schedule, but plan three evenly spaced meals over about a twelve-hour period. The goal is to eat only these three meals with nothing in between, so (for now) don't worry about how much you are eating—just focus on sticking to the three a day, not skipping any and not snacking in between. All food counts as snacks, and any beverage with significant calories also counts as a snack. If you have black coffee with a small amount of milk and no sugar mid-morning, don't worry about it, but a latte or a glass of wine should be considered a snack and is best to have with meals, not between.

Allow your body and mind at least a few days to get used to the new pattern. It may feel strange at first, but it gets easier once your body adapts. Your stomach will produce ghrelin surges at the times it normally expects food, so for the first few days of a different meal schedule you may feel transient hunger at the times you used to eat. Your body will quickly learn the new meal pattern, however, and those feelings will go away. If you are accustomed to eating every few hours, bear in mind that you may have to increase your meal size so that you can be satisfied for longer. Eating three miniature meals (instead of six miniature meals) is *not* healthy, habit-based weight loss. That's just dieting harder, and not a maintainable strategy.

Special circumstances may make you better suited to include a fourth feeding. If you exercise intensely after your evening meal, you may benefit from a shake or snack rather than going to bed without any post-workout nutrition. Also, if your work or personal schedule requires that you go seven or more hours between two meals, a feeding in the middle can help you get through that long period without building up an excessive appetite for the next meal or having to eat an uncomfortably large meal before to "make it through."

This situation often arises when people have lunch at noon and dinner at seven or eight p.m. If it's not possible to have lunch a little later, that means a long time between meals. Clients in this scenario often feel that they have to choose between two undesirable options: either eating an uncomfortable volume of food at midday to get to dinner, or eating a reasonable lunch but feeling starved by the time dinner rolls around. Getting overly full isn't comfortable, but getting overly hungry typically leads to munching while cooking or overeating when they finally get to their meal. Planning to eat something around three or four p.m. is very helpful in this case. However, to prevent adding excessive calories and preventing weight loss with the additional fourth meal, we make sure:

1. That lunch is appropriately sized so they are hungry for the midafternoon feeding.

2. That the midafternoon meal is sized to allow for hunger to return before dinner.

So, if you plan a fourth meal or snack to bridge the gap between two other meals that are seven or more hours apart, keep in mind that you don't need the snack or preceding meal to be very large. Your next meal is only a few hours away.

Last, if your schedule varies day to day or you have a different pattern on weekends, it's okay to have three meals some days and four meals others. Many people don't get up as early on weekends as they do during the week, so they find three meals works best for Saturday and Sunday, even if a longer waking time makes four meals better suited for Monday through Friday.

WHY IT'S WORTH IT

Satisfaction is key to the success and longevity of any nutrition plan, and this habit is going to help you form a pattern of eating that is as physically satisfying as possible.

TESTIMONIAL

"I think this habit has helped me to realize that I don't need to carry around all of this extra food with me in my lunch bag to work and then feel obligated to eat it just because I think I'm supposed to eat six times a day. That was likely contributing to overeating."

(Three cheers for being satisfied!) Most people can rely on willpower to temporarily stick to a program that doesn't satisfy their appetite—but not for a lifetime. Eating three satisfying meals, with no snacking in between (and no mini-meals!), helps you lose fat without having to be hungry all the time. Best of all, you can eat until you are actually satisfied, a concept which to many dieters seems like a distant memory. When all your food is concentrated into meals, with no snacks or impulse bites between, you can sit down to a full plate of food, get comfortably satisfied and still achieve a calorie level low enough to help you lose fat. Research shows that between-meal snacking, even on "healthy" foods like yogurt and fruit, can add up to excess calories without improving satiety. So avoiding snacks and having more filling meals is a great place to start getting more satisfied.

> EATING THREE SATISFYING MEALS, WITH NO SNACKING IN BETWEEN (AND NO MINI-MEALS!), HELPS YOU LOSE FAT WITHOUT HAVING TO BE HUNGRY ALL THE TIME. BEST OF ALL, YOU CAN EAT UNTIL YOU ARE ACTUALLY SATISFIED, A CONCEPT WHICH TO MANY DIETERS SEEMS LIKE A DISTANT MEMORY.

HOW IT WORKS

You already know that fat loss requires consuming fewer calories than you burn. Yet most dieters find that reducing calorie intake leads to decreased feelings of satisfaction and increased hunger. These sensations can make us pretty uncomfortable. My goal as a coach has always been to help my clients achieve that calorie deficit in the most comfortable way possible. The experience of losing fat doesn't have to be all that bad!

People trying to control calorie intake often fall into a pattern of eating lots of small meals throughout the day, so they don't have to go long periods without food. Or, they might set out to eat small, low-calorie meals (like a salad with chicken breast and low-fat dressing) but end up hungry just an hour or two later and steal three mini Kit Kat bars from their coworker's candy drawer, or raid their grocery bags on the drive home, and by the time they pull into the driveway, they've eaten four cups of bagged popcorn. Trying to eat meals that are *too small* is one of the easiest ways to go wrong in weight loss.

Eating six small meals per day used to be popular advice for weight loss, until research started to show that it didn't have any benefits. We've all heard trainers tell us to "stoke the fire of our metabolism" by eating often, but this has been debunked by scientific study. You don't burn any more calories by eating frequently. Eating many small meals backfires for many people because they end up eating enough calories to maintain their weight if you add them all up. Research reveals that the more frequently people eat, the higher their total calorie intake tends to be. As studies have been amassed using different populations and different diet prescriptions and meal patterns, it's become increasingly apparent that there is zero metabolic or satiety advantage to eating six times a day versus three times a day. Whether you call eating incidents meals or snacks is inconsequential.

EATING MANY SMALL MEALS BACKFIRES FOR MANY PEOPLE BECAUSE THEY END UP EATING ENOUGH CALORIES TO MAINTAIN THEIR WEIGHT IF YOU ADD THEM ALL UP. RESEARCH REVEALS THAT THE MORE FREQUENTLY PEOPLE EAT, THE HIGHER THEIR TOTAL CALORIE INTAKE TENDS TO BE.

A 2011 paper in the *Journal of Nutrition* observes findings on eating between meals, explaining why it promotes weight gain: "The energy content of snacks was never compensated for at the next meal and led consistently to a positive energy balance compared with no-snack conditions. Biologically, the snack-induced insulin secretion suppressed the late increase in plasma FFA (Free Fatty Acids), which may have contributed to the inhibition of satiety."

A study published in 2012 investigated the impact of meal frequency on appetite and hunger by providing two groups of men with the same amount of food, but divided into three meals or fourteen meals. Throughout the day, blood samples were collected to analyze hunger-related hormones, and subjects answered questions about their hunger and fullness. The three-meal pattern was significantly more satisfying, with men reporting less hunger and more fullness throughout the day. Blood samples showed that levels of the hunger hormone ghrelin were significantly reduced by eating three times per day, and blood sugar was lower over the total course of the 24 hours, which is also favorable for metabolic health. If the subjects got the same total amount of food though, why wasn't hunger equally satisfied when it was given in many little meals? One of the researchers explained that when meals are too small, they simply don't cause enough of a hormonal stimulus to fully "turn off" hunger: "The differential responses between smaller and larger eating occasions may simply be due to the inability of the body to detect the size of a smaller eating occasion as an adequate physiological load, reducing or eliminating the eating-related responses typically observed when larger eating occasions occur."

Frequent eating doesn't provide any extra metabolic benefit. It leads to higher calorie intake, and provides less satisfaction than three meals. Doesn't sound so promising for weight loss, does it?

TESTIMONIAL

"I learned that eating well three times a day not only fits my busy lifestyle, but I actually feel better both physically and mentally. And I am not going to starve if I don't snack and wait five hours between meals. Now, I can zero in on listening to my body. I like to think of it as becoming closer to myself and getting to know me better. That is empowering."

A study published in August 2013 found that consuming high-sugar, high-fat snacks between meals not only caused weight gain but also decreased serotonin transporter activity in the hypothalamus, a region of the brain known to be involved in body weight regulation. Adding the same exact high-fat, high-sugar foods to the main three meals of the day, however, did not cause the same changes in neurotransmitter activity.

Although we know that serotonin plays a role in weight maintenance, more research is needed to clarify the precise impact of decreased serotonin activity that may occur with snacking between meals. It seems clear, though, that snacking between meals causes different neurotransmitter signaling changes compared to simply eating more food at meals.

TESTIMONIAL

"For me, it's more than just a reduced sweet tooth. It's elimination of the sugar binging. For me, sugar begets sugar. So even though I've had some dark chocolate at the end of a meal a few times, I haven't felt the need to binge, and I haven't had the need to have something sweet every evening. Huge win for me, control over sugar!! Yeah!"

While people in research studies can help us learn more about the biological effects on appetite, there's a real-world practicality to be considered too: the amount of effort it takes to follow a meal pattern. Most people who have tried to stick to a plan of small frequent meals know that while there's something *nice* about being able to eat more often, it requires a constant effort to keep to restricted portions. We can't go unsatisfied or partially satisfied perpetually. The difficulty of constant restraint and never feeling truly satisfied often trigger episodes of rebound overeating, or at the very least, a growing sense of discontent and resentment. I don't want to stop eating at "80 percent full," as one popular weight-loss adage instructs. I don't want to go through life sub-satisfied in any way, come to think of it. That sounds like a pretty raw deal.

Have you ever thought you are "too hungry" for your own good? Have you suspected that maybe you have a miscalibrated meter somewhere inside that makes your body want more food than it seems to need? If so, listen up: having three or four satisfying meals also can help "reset" your hunger and fullness cues. Research suggests that three or four eating episodes per day without snacking leads to a metabolic shift toward burning more fat and relying less on carbohydrates. This metabolic shift further decreases appetite and helps to repair symptoms of glucose instability caused by metabolic inflexibility.

HAVING THREE OR FOUR SATISFYING MEALS ALSO CAN HELP "RESET" YOUR HUNGER AND FULLNESS CUES. RESEARCH SUGGESTS THAT THREE OR FOUR EATING EPISODES PER DAY WITHOUT SNACKING LEADS TO A METABOLIC SHIFT TOWARD BURNING MORE FAT AND RELYING LESS ON CARBOHYDRATES.

What does that mean? You are likely to be metabolically inflexible if you experience hypoglycemia, sudden feelings of needing to eat *now*, and swift bouts of dizziness, nausea, cold or crankiness if a meal is delayed. Your body has two main fuels, carbohydrates and fat, and a healthy metabolism can readily switch between the two depending on fuel availability. The unpleasant symptoms mentioned above arise from your body suddenly running short of fuel, and they occur if your physiology has adjusted to preferring carbohydrates and has a harder time adjusting to burning fatty acids. Mastering this habit by eating three or four meals per day can actually help to improve these symptoms by helping your body stay flexible to fuels, readily burning fat or carbohydrates depending on your needs.

TESTIMONIAL
"I learned how much mental space is freed up to think about life instead of hunger."

Less frequent eating improves your ability to burn fat because it allows for long enough intervals between meals while you're in a fasting state. If you eat often, you never get into this state. In the fasting state, after you've assimilated the fuels from your last meal, your body turns from absorbing and storing fuels into using stored fuels. During this time (typically three to five hours after you last ate) is when your body switches on its fat-mobilizing and fat-burning processes. Your muscles and liver, which comprise a sizable segment of your metabolically active tissue, both switch from using carbohydrates to using stored fat as fuel. This transition away from relying on glucose is an adaptation that keeps your blood sugar steady, as glucose slowly released from stores in the liver is available for the brain to use.

If you suffer from episodes of hypoglycemia or low blood sugar on a regular basis, your muscles and liver may not be efficiently making this switch to oxidizing fat as well as they could. The solution: gradually train your body to go longer between meals so it improves its ability to burn fat for fuel.

Eating between meals, or eating again in less than three hours (interrupting the body's approach of the fasting state), shifts your metabolism back toward carbohydrate burning, priming you to store excess calories ingested as body fat, as opposed to burning them off. In fact, measurement of a person's RQ (respiratory quotient, the ratio of carbohydrate to fat burning) is highly predictive of their risk for obesity. The key here: the more carbohydrates you are burning, the more readily you store fat. When you get several intervals during the day of fasting for five or more hours, you burn more fat, your blood sugar doesn't crash and hunger doesn't come upon you like a destructive tidal wave. It behaves more like a gently rising tide.

TESTIMONIAL

"I am frankly amazed at how my cravings to eat between meals have virtually disappeared. I've always fought with that and just doing this one habit has fixed that problem completely! My moods also feel more even. And yes, the hunger being less of an emergency—wow! It just kind of creeps up slowly instead of bam, I'm starving!"

Enhanced fat oxidation is a powerful metabolic tool in getting lean, but let's not overlook the logistical benefits too—fewer meals per day requires less planning, less thinking about food and fewer dishes to wash. I did the cooler and Tupperware thing for years. It was only after I *stopped* that I realized how much effort I saved by not having to pack up and carry three "meals" to work, and how much more productive I became with less hunger distracting me and fewer breaks for food. Being freed from washing a mountain of plastic containers also added precious free time to my day to do things I enjoy.

Additionally, letting yourself get fully hungry between meals increases your sensitivity to leptin, a hormone that helps to naturally promote leanness, decrease appetite and promote energy expenditure. Maintaining leptin sensitivity is associated with maintaining your weight loss for the rest of your life. People who decrease their leptin sensitivity (through yo-yo dieting, high fat intake, inadequate sleep or other factors) are more likely to regain weight they lost and gain weight slowly as they age.

You might be tempted to think that eating only once or twice a day might therefore be even better than having three or four meals. However, research also shows that eating less than three meals isn't optimal. People who eat only one or two meals a day have been shown to have higher body fat levels than those who eat three times daily, and controlled feeding studies have concluded that eating fewer than three times per day results in poorer appetite control.

RESEARCH SUPPORTS THAT THE SWEET SPOT FOR OPTIMAL APPETITE CONTROL AND MOST COMFORTABLE FAT LOSS IS EATING THREE OR FOUR TIMES PER DAY—NOT MORE, NOT LESS.

Among my clients, I've observed several people try to make a two-meals-per-day plan work, but in most cases it does not. Typically, a person can initially stick to a calorie deficit eating two meals, but after a day or two their meals tend to creep upward in size until the person is in calorie balance again, and not losing weight. The physical and psychological stress of extended fasts on a daily basis, as well as the liver glycogen depletion that occurs, may be mechanisms behind why two meals a day just doesn't help most people to lose weight and maintain athletic capacity (even if the individuals do like it for simplicity).

Research supports that the sweet spot for optimal appetite control and most comfortable fat loss is eating three or four times per day—not more, not less.

WHAT TO EXPECT

Having taught this habit to hundreds of clients, I can give you a preview of the experience that often unfolds. In the first week, you may experience:

- Shock at how frequently you used to eat
- Surprise as you catch yourself automatically eating between meals (If this happens, just stop and correct yourself.)
- Feelings of freedom and independence as you learn you don't need to carry food with you everywhere you go
- The realization that you need to eat more substantial meals to make it four to six hours until your next feeding
- Glee at enjoying substantial meals for the first time in a long time (if you're a chronic dieter)
- A reduced sweet tooth
- Improved blood sugar stability as your body adapts to using fat between meals
- Less hunger that feels like an emergency
- An increasing awareness of yourself, your thoughts and possibly things that you used to snack on to avoid thinking about or feeling hunger
- New non-food routines for evening entertainment, unwinding rituals after work and alleviating boredom

Update your habit tracker with the following Lean Habit, "Eat 3 or 4 meals without snacking in between," and get started with tracking your first behavioral goal!

HABIT	1	2	3	4	5	6	7	8	9	10	11	12	13	14
Eat 3 or 4 meals without snacking														

LEAN HABIT 2:
MASTER YOUR HUNGER

WHAT TO DO

Commit to feeling steady hunger for 30 to 60 minutes before each meal. If you've been ignoring your appetite cues for years, you might need some practice to get accustomed to feeling them again. Here are some tips on recognizing genuine body hunger and distinguishing it from false hunger (emotional or mental appetite).

- Real hunger builds gradually, and may go through an initial phase of coming and going before becoming a steady sensation.

- False hunger or a desire to eat may arise suddenly and doesn't last for more than about 20 to 30 minutes. This is because it is generally triggered by an emotion, time of day, smelling or seeing an appetizing food or viewing an advertisement—not a genuine bodily need.

- If you aren't sure whether you're feeling genuine body hunger or a false hunger, simply take a 20- to 30-minute wait-and-see period.

It may be helpful to remind yourself that hunger is not an emergency, and that feeling appropriately hungry for each meal is your assurance that you're eating just the right amount for fat loss. Your body is well equipped to get through long periods of time without food—weeks, in fact.

So don't panic at the first sign of hunger. Instead, think of it in the same way as when you notice you feel tired in the evening. Feeling tired isn't a sign that something is wrong that must be addressed immediately, it's simply a signal from your body to remind you gently that it's ready for sleep. Nothing bad happens when you get tired for a while, just like nothing harmful happens when you get hungry for a while. You aren't going to face sleep deprivation or starvation by feeling either sensation for a moderate amount of time. These signals are just information, wisdom from within.

IT MAY BE HELPFUL TO REMIND YOURSELF THAT HUNGER IS NOT AN EMERGENCY, AND THAT FEELING APPROPRIATELY HUNGRY FOR EACH MEAL IS YOUR ASSURANCE THAT YOU'RE EATING JUST THE RIGHT AMOUNT FOR FAT LOSS.

Feeling genuine physical hunger is favorable; hunger should reassure you that you are on the right track for weight loss if you feel it for at least 30 minutes before eating every time. Likewise, even the absence of hunger is a signal to heed: if you aren't feeling physical hunger as described above, you are receiving valid direction that you shouldn't be eating.

If your job, like many people's, involves set times of availability to eat, such as an inflexible lunch break, do your best to reverse-engineer your preceding meal size so you get hungry at about the right time, half an hour or an hour before your lunch break. That means experimenting with how much breakfast works for you.

If you are tempted to eat to prevent hunger because you could potentially end up being hungry for *hours and hours* (for example, if you're a surgeon going into an eight-hour operation), weigh the options of eating before versus eating after. The drawbacks of eating beforehand, when not hungry include possibly exceeding your calorie needs, but the drawbacks of not eating beforehand include possibly having to be hungry for a number of hours. Being hungry for that long may result in poorer decision making and overeating when you do eat your next meal. There's no clear winner, so I suggest predicting how many hours you'd have to be hungry, assessing your own tolerance for hunger and just picking one. If you're going to be out running errands for 45 minutes, though, there is absolutely no need to prevent hunger by eating beforehand if you aren't hungry yet. Engaging in hunger prevention on a regular basis ends up becoming weight-loss prevention, so you want to avoid it when possible.

If the urge to eat arises frequently when you know you aren't truly hungry, don't blame yourself, just try to understand what it is you really want. It might be that you're seeking emotional healing, comfort, fun or connection with someone else. Go get that thing. You deserve it, and you don't have to settle for food when you really crave fun, love or some relaxation.

Many of our clients find that practicing this habit feels incredibly empowering and increases the enjoyment of every meal. Not to mention, it can be the kick in the pants we need to recognize other unmet needs we have—and start meeting them instead of using food as a surrogate.

WHY IT'S WORTH IT

What if I told you that your body is already equipped with a marvelously accurate system for monitoring your energy intake and expenditure, and using this system properly will help you find the right amount of food? You might not believe me. And if you did believe me, you would likely begin to wonder why you've spent endless hours of your life counting calories or tallying points to determine how much food to eat.

Sadly, most dieters don't think of their body as being helpful to them in their weight-loss journey. It's a lot more common to view body signals like hunger as our foes. How many times have you felt like your hunger was a beast you were doing battle against, or an enemy you were always trying to keep at bay, knowing that despite your best efforts—darn it—it would come back?

Believe it or not, having hunger is a good thing. It's time you became friends with your hunger. That your body gives you a hunger signal is helpful, in fact; it can help you gauge how your energy intake is stacking up against your expenditure, reassuring you that you are on track or giving you hints that you need to adjust for better results.

Mastering your hunger involves learning just how hungry you should feel and when. As you practice this habit, know that it is completely normal and absolutely okay if you discover you have some fear or anxiety associated with hunger. Many of my clients do, and I did as well. Working in safe, small steps, it is possible to let the fear and anxiety go, enjoy a better relationship with your body and have an easier time shedding weight.

MASTERING YOUR HUNGER INVOLVES LEARNING JUST HOW HUNGRY YOU SHOULD FEEL AND WHEN.

After all, hunger is a normal, healthy signal from the body, and we can't avoid it altogether and still lose fat. Practicing this habit will help you get into a calorie deficit without undereating by an unsafe margin, stressing yourself out or counting calories. And your hunger is going to help you do it.

HOW IT WORKS

If you can't remember the last time you felt physiological hunger, it's likely that you've been eating too much to lose weight. Eating "because it's time," for emotional reasons or to go along with social cues can prevent your weight-loss program from getting results because you don't get into the energy-deficit state. If you can recall a time when you ate abundantly for several days in a row—vacations often make good examples—you know that hunger can be totally absent for days or weeks at a time. We can go on enjoying ourselves, and if you enjoy food as much as I do, it's certainly no problem to keep eating even when hunger is nowhere in the picture—but that absence of hunger is a signal itself. It's one that we can hear and translate into a useful message. When we don't feel any hunger for long stretches of time (and we are perfectly healthy), we are likely eating above our energy needs. We don't need calorie-tracking software, we don't need to wait until our pants are tight or we get on the scale and see a 10-pound increase. We can hear our body's language and know what it means to get the "silent treatment" from our hunger. Even in its silence, it's looking out for us.

On the other hand, experiencing hunger for extended periods creates stress (both physical and emotional) and often leads to obsessing about food and eating, which can significantly reduce your quality of life. Furthermore, going through a long stretch of being overly hungry (deliberately or not) is a common trigger for overeating or binge eating after food becomes available again. This is one of the reasons why binge eating is prevalent among figure competitors who attain very low body fat levels by adhering to a strict diet before a show. "Cutting" body fat by extreme dieting requires an enormous amount of willpower and hunger tolerance; in the weeks before stepping onstage, competitors are fighting hunger nearly 24 hours a day. After the competition, however, many competitors are afflicted by what feels like a scary loss of control over their eating, and binges can continue for months, quickly adding 10 or 20 pounds of fat to the person's previously ultra-lean frame. This isn't due to any fault of the individual; it's a powerful biological and psychological response to counteract the drastic energy shortage, rapid fat loss and mental strain created by the pre-contest diet. Feeling hunger before you eat is healthy and maintainable. Feeling hunger relentlessly around the clock is intolerable for very long.

RESEARCH HAS SHOWN THAT LEARNING TO CORRECTLY IDENTIFY THE SENSATION OF HUNGER AND DIFFERENTIATE IT FROM OTHER STIMULI ALLOWS PEOPLE TO NATURALLY REGULATE THEIR FOOD INTAKE, IMPROVE INSULIN SENSITIVITY AND LOSE WEIGHT.

Even if you could tolerate near-constant hunger, you would likely be eating too little to support optimal workouts and maintain (or increase) lean mass. It's just not necessary to feel hunger hour after hour to get lean and healthy. There are no points awarded for suffering. If your calorie intake is too low, your hunger is going to help give you the message. It will wake you at night, occupy your entire afternoon and generally not leave you alone.

Luckily, research has shown that learning to correctly identify the sensation of hunger and differentiate it from other stimuli allows people to naturally regulate their food intake, improve insulin sensitivity and lose weight. How well does it work? A 2010 study reported that after receiving training to identify hunger and eat in response to hunger only, overweight subjects lost an average of 15 pounds in five months.

How it works is simple: eating only when we are truly hungry reduces calorie intake because it helps us skip the calories that our body doesn't need. Aside from weight loss, moving away from non-hunger-driven eating can be the nudge we need to develop healthier and more effective strategies to relax, de-stress or manage emotions. If mindless munching has been a crutch to cope with excessive stress or avoid problems, taking steps to change your eating pattern might have a very juicy payoff in helping you face and deal with problems directly.

WHAT HUNGER *IS*, AND WHAT IT *ISN'T*

When I discuss this habit with clients, I ask them to describe what hunger feels like and where they feel it in their body. It's important that I make sure you're clear on what I mean when I suggest feeling hunger at regular intervals as a habit. It's not like arithmetic or the capital of Kansas; schools don't teach all second graders what hunger feels like and how to distinguish it from thirst, sadness or nausea. You have probably had to piece together your definition of hunger from experience and hearing clues from other people.

While everyone's description is a little different, the important thing I'm looking for is **a belly-centered sensation.** And most people actually do say something like "a grumbling stomach" or "a gnawing sensation in my abdomen," but the occasional client will define hunger as a headache, sleepiness or mouth feeling like "wanting something to crunch on." In these cases, it's worth clarifying that these sensations are valid, and may indicate a need or desire for something else, but they are not hunger. Headaches, sleepiness or wanting to crunch on something are not reliable indicators of a need for fuel. Hunger is felt in the stomach; my favorite definition is "an empty-hollow sensation in the abdomen, which may or may not be accompanied by muscular contractions or growling."

Physical sensations that are not actually *hunger* can be mistaken for it, leading to unnecessary eating. Similarly, social cues, routine or boredom are some of the most common reasons people eat when they aren't hungry. As Mario Ciampolini writes in a 2013 research report in the *International Journal of General Medicine*: "Stimuli that are not influenced by food intake may override or obscure hunger and include compelling extrinsic factors such as highly palatable and heavily marketed food, social factors such as eating in the presence of others, and intrinsic factors such as emotions. Furthermore, people often interpret a wide range of nonspecific body sensations as 'hunger.' These sensations, poorly identified as an undifferentiated unpleasant feeling, could include nausea, pain, or thirst. They can be particularly confusing since they may temporarily disappear after food intake giving the false notion that they represent hunger."

Another commonly cited reason for eating in the absence of hunger is to *prevent hunger.* Before going into a three-hour meeting, many people will be tempted to grab a snack bar from their desk just so that they don't get hungry during the meeting. Preventing hunger, however, prevents weight loss. It's okay to feel hunger, and if you want to lose weight, feeling some hunger is necessary. It won't harm you.

SCALING HUNGER MASTERY

Everyone feels hunger differently before eating. If feeling hungry for 30 to 60 minutes before each time you eat seems too hard to start with, that's okay. You can practice just making sure you feel genuine physical hunger for 10 or 15 minutes before you eat, which still means not eating out of boredom, stress or routine. Eating only when you're hungry is the number one lifelong skill you can learn for leanness, and in forming a healthy relationship with food. If you need time to nail this, take the time. It is worth it.

Note that if you customarily go more than 60 minutes of feeling hunger and not eating, your necessary skill will be to stop doing that to yourself. If you have to plan differently or adjust so that you can meet your body's needs for fuel, that is an important behavioral change for leanness too. Many people I have worked with over the years got so busy working, running around on weekends or caring for their children that they put their own needs last and ignored hunger for several hours on a regular basis. No wonder they overate when the next meal was finally in front of them!

DRAMA DECREASING LINGO TIP:

You're Not Starving, You're Just Hungry.

Our language has profound impact on how we feel. I recommend that unless you have been without food for more than a week you try to avoid saying, "I'm starving." Even thinking those words has a way of making things feel more urgent than they really are. More truthfully, you'd say, "I'm hungry." You might say you are "very hungry" or "uncomfortably hungry," perhaps, but let's be honest—you aren't starving. You are in no danger. Speaking accurately and being aware of your thoughts to avoid melodrama can go a long way to making weight loss easier.

"BUT I HATE HUNGER!!"

I was terrified of hunger for most of my life. I absolutely hated it. And in retrospect, it's crystal clear that my hunger-hating mind-set contributed to my difficulty getting below a certain body-fat percentage and weight. I was preventing hunger all the time with snacks and packed meals and food stashed in the car, my gym bag, my work desk ... and actually preventing myself from getting into the calorie deficit I needed to lose those last few stubborn pounds. After recovery in my teens from a restrictive eating disorder, during which I felt constant hunger alongside other painful emotions and depression, I was terrified that feeling hunger meant "going back there" to a dark, unhappy, painful place. I had associated being hungry with the most painful time of my life—and it led to me dodging hunger at all costs, remaining fearful of it because I never had to experience it, and maintaining a softer body than I wanted.

It was actually my husband, Roland, who gently nudged me to experience just a bit of hunger, noting how I habitually treated hunger as if it were a flesh-eating virus, preventing it as much as possible and suffering greatly when I was afflicted. In addition to being the love of my life, Roland too is a professional nutrition coach, so I had two good reasons to listen to his advice. I admit, though, that I was *incredibly resistant* to the idea. While my logical brain agreed that being hungry for a little while before eating was good advice, my emotional brain wanted to run in the other direction (and bring a snack in case I'd be gone a while). But with his gentle way of suggesting with absolutely no pressure, Roland convinced me to make an attempt. I decided to allow myself to feel hunger for a couple minutes a day without judging it, just see if it was actually nightmarish agony as I had built it up in my mind … or if it was really just a mild sensation. And the results of my experiment?

Without the fear and worry, hunger is really not that bad. It's not nearly as painful as some pairs of shoes I have worn willingly for entire days. It was just the emotions I had linked to hunger that were causing the real suffering.

I had tied hunger to anxiety, danger, self-deprivation, uncertainty, punishment and low self-esteem. Because when I suffered those emotions the most in my life, those were the days I was starving myself.

But the emotional associations didn't actually have anything to do with feeling hunger; it was only my experiences and memories that created that connection. You may also realize that it's not hunger you hate, but uncertainty, insecurity or feeling like you're missing out on pleasure. The good news is that you don't have to experience any of those things to feel hungry and manage your weight.

Compared to positive experiences, negative experiences leave more significant imprints in our memories, so if you have negative memories or associations with hunger, try to look between them to see if there are other times you felt hunger but it really wasn't so bad. On occasions when I've been engaged and having fun (like a really fun shopping spree!), I can remember being hungry for at least an hour or two, but because I was having fun, I wasn't bothered by it. If you practice feeling brief periods of hunger on your own terms when you know you're safe, happy and secure, you'll begin to dissociate all the unpleasant layers from it. It's just a sensation.

If you want to take it slow, please do. I'm timid. I get into a pool one inch at a time, and I made friends with hunger the same way: exceedingly slowly, and on my own terms. I didn't run to it and embrace in the middle of a field of wildflowers; I gave it a hesitant five-minute trial at a time. And I realized it wasn't so bad.

After letting myself feel hunger for a few minutes at a time on a regular basis, I started to see perks. I didn't have to play the game of "Am I eating too much? I think I'm eating too much …" because if my hunger was there before each meal, I had reassurance I was giving my body the right amount of food. Eventually I didn't want to eat without that reassurance. Learning to accept hunger and get past my fear of it showed me how helpful it is, and it's one of the key tools that helps me stay lean, year after year, without a lot of effort.

Eventually, eating when not hungry for 30 to 60 minutes beforehand seemed like putting on a raincoat when the sun was shining. It just wouldn't cross my mind. If food was offered, it wasn't a struggle to say, "No thanks, I don't really need that right now."

"PROCRASTINEATING" AND "EATERTAINMENT"

In my work with clients over the years, I've identified these two phenomena as a couple of the most common reasons that people eat when they aren't hungry. Procrastineating is, as you probably guessed, using food to put off working on a project or chore. Students commonly procrastineat when it's time to study for exams, working through bowls of popcorn or chips in tacit avoidance of the work that needs to get done. Getting started on a research paper or firing up TurboTax to tackle your taxes each April always seems like it would be better accomplished in a few minutes. *Right after I get a snack I'll get down to business.*

Procrastineating is not an indication that someone is lazy; it can be quite the opposite. It is surprisingly prevalent in hard-working, successful people who rarely (or never) give themselves permission to take a break during the workday. They work all day, then come home and face a stack of mail, a sink of dishes and three loads of laundry that need folding. And in that space between completing one hard work-shift at the office and beginning another stretch of work at home, procrastineating is persistent. If you keep continuous pressure on yourself to be productive every minute of every day, eating may be the one pause that seems valid enough. After all, it's a basic human need to *eat*. No one, not even ourselves, should give us grief over stopping to *eat*, right? That should be excusable even if there's no other way to stop working. So we do the only legitimate thing we know how to do to enjoy a few minutes where we don't have to work. We eat.

If that sounds like you, then while you practice Hunger Mastery, I encourage you to take other breaks. Let yourself have a few minutes of fresh air during the mid-afternoon grind, or take 10 minutes to lie down on the bed after work instead of seeing only two choices: eat or jump into chores right away. Rest breaks and rejuvenation *are* productive and valuable usage of your time. If you are hesitant to take 5 or 10 minutes "off," judging it as a waste, remember that you previously would have taken that time to snack, so it's equally (if not more) valid to use those minutes for calorie-free rejuvenation.

If you know you are prone to procrastination (and eating becomes a form of that), here are a few things to try:

First, make reasonable expectations of what you can do in a day. Blocking off six hours to study straight is just not realistic! Make a flexible schedule that isn't a big stretch, like 60- to 90-minute stretches of study/work time, with breaks in between so it looks easy to stick to, not intimidating. Picture how you'll feel at the end of the day if you stick to your intentions, or close to them, and how positive that experience will be.

When you stick to your plan, give yourself lots of praise. Pour it on. "Go me, I'm having lunch when I planned to!" "Go me, taking my 2:45 walk!" "Yeah, Laura! I just thought of going to grab a muffin but realized I'd rather get some water since I'm not really hungry!" "I rock!" And plan something fun to do at the end of the day, like Facebook surfing, browsing Pinterest, watching a television show or opening a book you're reading just for enjoyment. If the urge strikes to procrastinate by doing those things during the times you've planned to work, you can say, "Oh, I'll get to do that later."

Eatertainment is a word I use to describe eating to alleviate or prevent boredom, and it occurs in many forms. We can seek out food just because we have nothing else to do on a Saturday afternoon, or we can fall into the habit of automatically pairing food with other entertainment forms, like movies or the television, regardless of whether we are hungry or not. We can eatertain ourselves at a party if we don't know anyone to pass the time. We can even eatertain others when they are visiting us and we aren't sure how to make conversation or keep them occupied.

No one likes to be bored, and craving some stimulus is a natural human inclination. I'm not suggesting that you have to stop socializing over dinners out, or that it's somehow wrong to enjoy or look forward to your food if you want to lose weight. It will not slow your weight-loss progress at all to let delicious food add to the enjoyment of a leisurely evening. It's fine to linger over your Sunday morning eggs and toast while doing the crossword. I find food enjoyable too! But to prevent eatertainment from interfering with your fat-loss goals, bear Hunger Mastery in mind: if you are hungry for 30 to 60 minutes before each time you eat, you are still executing the critical habit. If you are eating in the absence of hunger just for fun, you are possibly preventing yourself from achieving a lean body. Also, keep in mind that consuming food while your attention is elsewhere makes it all-too-easy to eat more than you need to because you get distracted.

EATING A SANDWICH IN FRONT OF THE TELEVISION IS NO MORE FATTENING THAN EATING A SANDWICH IN A ZEN GARDEN WITH COMPLETE FOCUS ON EVERY BITE, BUT IF THE TELEVISION DISTRACTS YOU INTO EATING A SANDWICH, AND THEN SOME CHIPS, AND THEN SOME COOKIES AND FINALLY REALIZING YOU DIDN'T NEED ALL THAT FOOD, YOU CAN SEE HOW PAIRING FOOD WITH OTHER ENTERTAINMENT *CAN* BE A PROBLEM.

If you find yourself bored but not hungry, use other activities besides eating to occupy and engage yourself until your body needs food. Have other things that you can also do if you get bored; a puzzle, a book, checking your favorite websites, chatting with your spouse or calling a pal can all help meet your need for stimulation without food. And if you are intentionally pairing food with another activity, stay tuned in to how much you are eating by checking in periodically. Eating a sandwich in front of the television is no more fattening than eating a sandwich in a Zen garden with complete focus on every bite, but if the television distracts you into eating a sandwich, and then some chips, and then some cookies and finally realizing you didn't need all that food, you can see how pairing food with other entertainment *can* be a problem.

CHALLENGES YOU MAY ENCOUNTER AND TWO POTENTIAL EXCEPTIONS

No Morning Appetite

If you don't feel hunger within one to two hours of waking up, I first recommend you reduce evening eating, because it's the most common cause of MIA morning appetite. Start by reducing your last meal of day so that you are just starting to feel empty at the time you go to bed. You can also adjust the timing of your evening meal, making it earlier, if needed, to leave 12 hours of fasting before you wake the next morning. (So if you get up at 7 a.m., finish eating for the night at 7 p.m.) Many times that results in waking up eager to eat! However, some people just don't feel hunger after waking, even if they were hungry going to bed. If these two changes don't work, it's better to just eat a planned breakfast emphasizing protein within an hour of waking up and use Hunger Mastery to guide subsequent meals. Eating breakfast (even if you haven't felt true hunger yet) is preferable to not having any breakfast and tackling a ravenous appetite at midday when it does appear. First thing in the morning is one time it may be wisest to make an exception to waiting for hunger for 30 to 60 minutes.

Exercise Masking Hunger

Exercise, especially intense training, has a short-term appetite-suppressive effect. However, if you don't eat anything after a hard workout and wait for hunger to return, you may get overwhelmed by how forcefully it reappears. If you have a mild or moderate workout, you probably don't need to adjust your meal timing at all. And if you work up an appetite while training, no problem; you'll enjoy that post-workout meal. However, if you exercise at high intensity and find your appetite is nowhere in sight afterward, it may be a second time where it is better to make an exception to the rule and not wait to feel hunger for 30 to 60 minutes.

- If possible, eating a whole-food, solid meal with carbohydrates and protein within an hour of finishing your workout is best. Real foods are more nutritious and will keep your appetite satisfied for more hours than a shake or sports drink. Even if you aren't hungry, this is one time you might want to just eat anyway. (Remember to count it as one of your three to four meals.)

- If you don't feel like you *can* eat after a tough workout or run, I recommend drinking eight ounces of sports drink to get some easily digested carbohydrates into your body (15 grams) and eating your next meal as soon as it is comfortable to do so. Count the small amount of sports drink as part of your next meal.

Inflexible Schedule

I expect that you have commitments, appointments and other things in your life that make it impossible to eat just "whenever." I do too. To have your hunger arrive at a time that works for you, you'll want to adjust the meal *before* to be larger or smaller. If you have a fixed time for lunch, for example, you'll want to do some experimentation to find out what breakfast works out so that you feel 30 to 60 minutes of genuine stomach hunger (not three hours) before lunch and are not eating lunch without any hunger present "just because it's time." I call this reverse-engineering your hunger. If you have an early dinner date with pals, you might eat a smaller lunch that day to ensure that you feel 30 to 60 minutes of hunger beforehand. It's normal to go through some trial and error while figuring out which of your common meals results in your hunger returning in four, five or six hours, or even longer. There's no rush. If you undershoot or overshoot, that's a normal part of practicing and learning. Stay focused and keep working at it, and you'll keep getting better. And remember, it's just food; don't take it too seriously or stress out.

WHAT YOU CAN EXPECT IN THE FIRST TWO WEEKS:

In the first two weeks of this habit, you can expect to discover that hunger isn't incredibly difficult to tolerate for brief periods of time. Thirty to 60 minutes passes easily, especially when you are doing something. You'll also find it feels really good to wait until you're hungry to eat!

Here are real-life client experiences with Hunger Mastery:

"I've also come to realize how mindlessly I ate in the past, and how, obviously, those extra calories can add up. Now, I really think about whether or not I'm hungry, and if what I do decide to eat is what I really want, or what's just 'available.' I can wait longer now for the food(s) I really want. Not compromising feels pretty darned good!"

"I learned that I don't have to reach for a snack the second I get home from work. Cooking dinner, allowing hunger to build ... the anticipation of dinner was almost as good as eating it (almost). There was a time when I was scared to feel hungry, but I actually found if I turned towards the feeling, rather than just grabbing food immediately, it is not actually very scary at all. It's kind of counterintuitive, but I find if I accept, acknowledge and sit with a feeling my body is trying to give me, I don't feel scared or panicked. Instead, I appreciate how amazing and intuitive my body is and I can thank it for letting me know it requires nutrition. Then I, calmly and mindfully, nourish it."

"When I started getting cravings, I just realized I was tired and tried to take it down a notch. I also told myself it was just PMS talking and not to freak out about it. Pretty soon it progressed to real hunger so I ate something—pretty simple. I learned that not overreacting to cravings can make them easier to deal with!"

"I surprised myself how often I think about putting something in my mouth when it isn't mealtime. While not being perfect, I did both habits together, fairly well. I also learned to think through my schedule for the day better, so that I'm spacing the meals and having food available at the expected times. I also like the feel of hunger. Makes me think my body is pac-manning all of the fat cells away."

"I focused on the one meal I knew would be at a certain time/place for the day, like lunch with friends or dinner with family. Then I worked forward or backwards from there and planned my other two meals. I learned I can go about five hours between meals and feel true hunger. I have had great results with these first two habits. They fit me and I own them! Can't wait to see what the next habit is!"

"I learned that when I really focus and pay attention, eating three or four times a day and maintaining awareness of hunger is not really that difficult! And, I don't have to be borderline antisocial to practice them (i.e., can't eat this, can't eat that, must eat at certain time[s], etc.). The habits feel natural."

"Letting myself be hungry for 30 to 60 minutes until a meal is not as difficult as I thought it might be two weeks ago. So I'm confident that I am flexible and committed to this process of change."

"It went well for me to acknowledge hunger and then observe and decipher its development, and eventually move away from the clock and the 30- to 60-minute guideline to just feeling habitually when it was the right time to eat. This was much more manageable falling into the net of habit 1. Likewise, I will approach future habits as falling into the net of the previous ones."

Time to update your Habit Tracker, you're graduating to habit 2! Now you'll be tracking *both* habits, eating three to four meals per day and practicing Hunger Mastery at each of those meals.

HABIT	1	2	3	4	5	6	7	8	9	10	11	12	13	14
Eat 3 or 4 meals without snacking														
Hunger Mastery (hunger for 30–60 minutes before eating)														

LEAN HABIT 3:
EATING JUST ENOUGH

WHAT TO DO

As we covered in prior habits, you know already that you'll want to embrace hunger for 30 to 60 minutes before each meal, and eat three to four meals a day without snacking. These two habits have helped steer you toward eating for the right reasons, and at the right intervals. Now that you've made strides with why and how often to eat, we'll focus on how much. For fat loss, the goal is to **eat a sufficient amount to be reasonably comfortable, but not more than that**. You might want to read that a second time, because it's very important.

If you eat too little, you will not be reasonably comfortable after a meal, and you'll end up hungry for longer than 60 minutes before each meal. Eating too little leads to feelings of deprivation and increases your likelihood of snacking between meals or overeating later (most likely at night). As one client put it so perfectly, "It really irks me when I ration myself the 'correct' amount of sweet potato only to eat a doughnut at work a few hours later because I'm starving." As I said in the very first habit, miniature meals are not the goal. I want you to get satisfied, but not push past what you need to get satisfied.

There is a range of food amount that can leave you feeling reasonably comfortable. There's not one "magic" bite that defines the perfect stopping point, so don't stress yourself out trying to feel exactly where it is. In baseball, as long as the batter hits the ball somewhere between the white lines, it's a fair ball. Well, Eating Just Enough is similar in that there's a boundary on either side. You can eat too little (foul ball to the left), or too much (foul ball to the right), but there's a bit of room in between.

Check out the graph below. When you feel hungry and begin to eat, the hunger isn't gone for the first few bites. If you stopped there, before you were satisfied, you would not have eaten enough. You might find yourself lingering in the kitchen peeking in cabinets, or thinking incessantly about food and when you'll eat next. And you might not be able to get to your next meal without snacking.

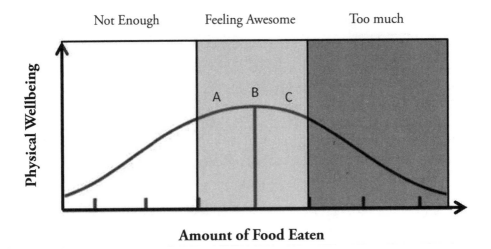

As you keep eating, hunger dissipates and you feel better up to a certain point, after which the positive physical sensations level off. In the middle zone, you don't feel any hunger and you also don't feel any pressure or heaviness from the food yet. You feel energetic and the food tastes the best. You feel satisfied, complete and like you could go for a brisk walk without asking for 10 minutes to digest first. If you stop eating in the middle zone, you shouldn't have any thoughts of food for at least one to two hours after eating. Eating past the middle zone doesn't make you feel any better though.

If you kept eating, you'd start to notice a bit of discomfort, a slight bloated sensation, a hint of pressure or heaviness in the abdomen or a sleepy feeling. These signs are indicators that you've crossed into the "too much" zone. And from there on, you just feel worse if you continue.

If you look at the letters A, B and C, those may be separated by only two or three bites in a meal. But at any point in that middle zone, you don't feel very different. It's all pretty good! So, even if you never eat all the way into the "too much" zone, if you aren't losing weight you may just need to fine-tune your stopping point. Stopping three bites earlier could move you from point C to B, or B to A, and get you out of maintenance and into weight loss. Just three bites.

WHY IT'S WORTH IT

As I've said before, fat loss comes down to creating an energy deficit. With the last habit, you've gotten some practice at identifying true hunger and allowing yourself to feel it for a period of time before you eat. Now we'll focus on the other side of the body's food-intake regulation system: the sensations that occur during eating that can guide you to the right place to put down the fork. Knowing how much to eat based on internal cues can help you take in the right amount of food, no matter where you are or what's on your plate.

You've probably had the experience of realizing too late that you ate more than you needed to. You may be able to recall specific nights when you had trouble falling asleep due to an overly full belly or really wanted to get home from a restaurant to put on stretchy pants. You may be all too familiar with the "Oh no. What have I done?" dread of noticing you ate far more popcorn at the movies than you intended to. Not only is it physically uncomfortable to eat too much, but it can set you back significantly in weight-loss progress to overeat even occasionally. And very important, it has a negative impact on our self-concept when we act in a way that is incongruent with our goals, and that lasts long after the extra calories have been burned off.

Even if you never, ever eat beyond comfortable satisfaction, if you aren't losing weight you're probably just a few bites away from your weight-loss zone. You could be only three bites past where you need to be for steady weight loss and, thanks to those three bites, you see nothing but maintenance—so close! (And so frustrating.) So let's hop to it and get this habit into your practice so you can start seeing results.

HOW IT WORKS

Try to bring more awareness to how you feel as you are eating. Try to stop once you reach satisfied (no longer hungry, not uncomfortable from eating too much). That's aiming for the "feeling awesome" zone (page 63).

If you're already losing weight just by thinking about stopping in the middle area and staying out of the "too much" zone, you're all set. However, if your weight loss is not progressing once you've been able to master that skill, you can move to the next level of refining this habit.

The more advanced level of Eating Just Enough is to slightly reduce your intake to see if you can remain relatively comfortable on three fewer bites of food at each meal. You may find that if you eat just a few bites less, you feel no different between meals and can achieve a calorie deficit needed for sustainable, comfortable weight loss. If your weight doesn't drop after you reduce by a small margin, make another small decrease in meal size (again, just a few bites) to find out if you can stay relatively comfortable on slightly fewer calories. As long as you can stay relatively comfortable, keep experimenting until weight loss starts.

Eating slowly, savoring each mouthful, taking small bites and chewing food thoroughly will all help you identify the feelings and sensations that occur as you eat and to recognize when you're getting satisfied. If you speed-eat, you'll miss your body's signals like road signs you blazed past at 100 mph.

Besides slowing down, another helpful tip is to accept that it's perfectly okay to not eat everything on your plate. Let your body guide you, instead of assuming that it takes a certain volume of food to be full. If you dine out, you are very likely to be served more than your body needs. Even at home, you may have developed the habit of dishing up more food onto your plate than Just Enough.

EATING SLOWLY, SAVORING EACH MOUTHFUL, TAKING SMALL BITES AND CHEWING FOOD THOROUGHLY WILL ALL HELP YOU IDENTIFY THE FEELINGS AND SENSATIONS THAT OCCUR AS YOU EAT AND TO RECOGNIZE WHEN YOU'RE GETTING SATISFIED.

Many of my clients initially report that they invariably clean their plates because they "hate to waste food." However, if the purpose of the food is to nourish you to greater health and be burned for energy, it's no less wasteful to eat unneeded food than it is to throw it in the trash or feed it to your dog. Either way, those bites of food that are above and beyond "just enough" are not getting burned for energy, nor are they helping you achieve great health. So, you can store it in your fat cells or let it be taken out with the trash, your pick. To reduce excess food ending up in either depot (your fat cells or the landfill), consider portioning just a bit less onto your plate, putting leftovers back in the fridge (even if it is only a bite or two) and asking for items to be left off your plate at restaurants if you know you probably won't eat them.

It can take a couple days to get a feel for how much is right for you, which is fine—be patient with yourself, as this skill is often not mastered quickly. Soon you'll reap the benefits as you tune in to your body signals.

It gets easier every time you practice. Many of our clients find that they initially liked feeling somewhat overfull, that the sleepy, numb feeling of a very full belly was appealing … until they got out of the habit of eating so much. After a few weeks of eating a more appropriate amount, eating to more than "just satisfied" feels lousy and undesirable.

There is a word in Swedish that doesn't translate directly into English, and that's a shame because it's ideal for describing the concept of Eating Just Enough. The word is *lagom,* and it indicates balance, sufficiency, "enough to go around," "not too much or too little" or "just right." It's not a word specific to describing food or eating; lagom could be used to describe someone's height, the weather or the firmness of a handshake. Lagom is more than just another vocabulary word though. I've been told it's an overarching value of the Swedish culture itself: the value and comfort of having enough, without excess.

Trying to clumsily translate it into English loses some of the appeal inherent in eating lagom. Eating a "sufficient" or "just what's necessary" amount implies a bit of scarcity and sounds a bit … well, I think it sounds dull or lacking. But eating lagom, to a Swede anyway, carries the connotation of appropriateness and comfort with an amount that is necessary without excess. So in addition to the bits of Swedish you may have learned while furnishing your past apartment at IKEA, carrying the word *lagom* in your mind is a helpful concept when framing your ideas of how much to eat.

Recap:

- If you tend to eat until you are overfull every day or even a few times a week, make your first goal to practice stopping at satisfied.

- If you never eat until overfull and are already stopping at satisfied but your weight is not decreasing, practice eating three bites less at each meal. You can accomplish that by serving yourself slightly less to start with, or leaving a few bites on the plate at the end of your meal (or slipping your dog three bites during the meal).

MIND OVER MATTER: MENTAL NINJA TIP

Much like hunger, our expectations are often much more dramatic (for the worse) than the reality of what it feels like to actually eat just a few bites less per day.

If you feel apprehensive about trying to eat a little less, sit with that fear and consider what you're afraid of. Are you afraid of your energy plummeting dramatically and being unable to perform your job? Are you afraid of passing out behind the wheel and causing a 10-car pileup on the freeway?

Needless to say, these extreme fears are exceedingly unlikely to happen, especially when you experiment with decreasing your intake in very small steps. If the amount of food you currently eat is totally comfortable, eating just a tiny bit less is not going to cause drastic and massive suffering. You can always carry an emergency snack with you in case your experiment leads to feeling unreasonably uncomfortable and you absolutely can't bear the hunger.

What's more likely to happen: you'll either feel no detectable difference, or you'll feel hunger arrive just a bit earlier but see that it's (surprisingly) totally manageable. Reassure yourself that you're fine; feeling some hunger before your next meal is an essential signpost, a positive signal confirming that you're getting closer to fat loss.

SKIRTING THE SAND TRAPS: VACATIONS AND PARTIES

If forging good nutrition habits and getting the body you want are a mini golf course, you can think of your day-to-day at-home routine as nice rolling green stretches of AstroTurf. But, of course, to keep things interesting there is a sand trap here and there that you could get mired in, a plastic rhinoceros to steer around and a giant windmill in between you and your goal. Not every day or every situation is equally easy to roll through. Let's review some of the obstacles to Eating Just Enough and some ways to manage each.

VACATION

Contrary to what your margarita-influenced brain might suggest, calories do in fact accumulate and count, regardless of whether you are in Tahiti or Detroit. You know this, I'm sure, but it's really easy to let your intentions relax and let yourself morph into thinking that overeating will somehow make the experience better. Spoiler alert: you don't get any more relaxed or rejuvenated by having tight pants on the flight home. In fact, I think coming home well aware of some newfound poundage only adds to the distress of heading back to work!

I'm not saying that there's anything wrong with going away and gaining 10 pounds, if you want to do that. But if you want to practice maintaining or continuing to lose weight even while away, it's absolutely feasible to continue your habits and still have a great time. Eat Just Enough is one of the essential habits I recommend for traveling, because it allows for the freedom to enjoy the French bread and artisan cheese in Paris, savor the wine and fettuccini in Italy or sink your teeth into a true Chicago pizza. Vacationing often means enjoying some special or regional cuisine that is more calorie-dense than your normal meals. However, if you accept that you don't have to eat it all (and it doesn't add much to the experience to eat past a certain point), you might surprise yourself that even eating "less healthy" foods puts hardly a dent in your progress. Don't be afraid to leave food on your plate, and remind yourself that you're vacationing primarily for fun, adventure or relaxation, and eating larger portions of food doesn't necessarily increase any of those rewards.

PARTIES

Whether it's a birthday celebration, holiday bash or girls' night, festive get-togethers can pose a challenge when you are practicing the habit of Eating Just Enough. It's easy to lose track of how full you're getting when there are many people to talk to. Popping bites of cheese and crackers in your mouth can help you maintain a comfortable conversational pace, without awkwardly lengthy pauses or feeling you're grilling someone with rapid-fire questions. If there is a large spread of food, it's tempting to try to taste everything, even if you're already satisfied. If you don't know anyone there and are feeling awkward or bored, it's very challenging to not eaertain yourself from start to finish! And many parties come with taste-bud-tempting seasonal fare: Christmas cookies, Super Bowl nachos, birthday cake or Easter candy.

Similar to vacation scenarios, you can successfully Eat Just Enough at parties by staying in the right frame of mind. First, remember (again) that more food isn't more fun. I've never heard anyone say, "I was pretty bored, honestly, but then once I got through that third helping of Buffalo wings, I'm having a much better time!" Second, commit to eating in "one act" instead of picking at things all night while standing around. It's impossible for your body to sense incoming calories and feel proportionately satisfied when they are trickled in over the course of an evening. Third, position yourself wisely in the venue. Hanging in the kitchen at a house party usually means staring down food all night long. Why not check out what's going on in the living room conversations or chat with the people gathered on the patio? If seats are not assigned at a wedding reception, sit with your back to the buffet and you'll find it's much, much easier to avoid going back for more. And regardless of the event, time on the dance floor is generally free of food temptations, so the more time you spend there, the better!

Rather than tasting everything and making multiple trips through the food, scan all the food items and put together one plate of the things you want most. Then, sit down somewhere (if possible) and enjoy it. Once you've gotten satisfied, think of yourself as being "fed" and done with eating. This can be a good time to have a pack of gum or mint handy to clean your palate, freshen your breath and prevent nibbling. Shift your focus back to talking with people, dancing, listening and having a good time. Needless to say, keeping your alcohol intake low or moderate will help prevent forgetting your plans and finding yourself halfway through a gigantic bowl of chips later.

CRAP. I OVERATE. NOW WHAT?

Succinctly stated, the best thing to do after you overeat is wait until you're hungry again to eat. Even if you drastically overdid it, you haven't permanently obliterated your appetite. It will return. When it does, let yourself feel hunger for 30 to 60 minutes, then eat. And keep rolling along, practicing your habits. That's all.

It's tempting to make it more complicated than that though. Before working with me, most of my clients had developed a habit of reacting to overeating with a complicated barrage of responses, including blaming themselves (or others), guilt-wallowing, regretting, restricting their food, compulsively exercising in penance and so forth. Occasionally, the spreadsheets came out, as they launched into diet mode and planned out two weeks of low-fat, low-carb meals. You may have done this yourself, feeling like you should compensate for the overeating incident, make up for it or perform some ritual to alleviate the guilt or shame you feel.

Focusing on feeling bad after you overeat doesn't help. Guilt trips don't burn any calories. They just make you feel like crap. And odds are when you feel like crap, and you think it's your fault that you feel like crap, you don't take the best care of yourself. Which can lead to the king of dieter's ironies: eating more because you feel bad about overeating. If you feel bad about overeating and your instinct is to overeat when you feel bad, you get trapped in a fattening whirlpool of despair. In an upcoming section I'll cover how to manage negative emotions in life without food, but in this scenario, you can escape the whirlpool by opting to not feel bad after you overeat. There is no need for negative emotions simply because you exceeded your calorie needs in the past. You can make healthy choices today and keep practicing the habits.

If your eyebrows raised reading that last part, you may feel instinctively resistant to applying that much kindness to yourself.

If you find yourself having a hard time letting go of guilt, it can be helpful to know that you're not being silly and are actually clinging to it for a very good reason. If you perceive value to something, it's tough to throw it away. (You may have found that out last time you tried to do some spring-cleaning or clear out your closet.) It's easy to believe that making yourself feel guilty will help you reach your goals by preventing you from doing the unwanted behavior, in this case overeating, again. So you may not take too easily to letting yourself off the hook.

The purpose of guilt as an emotion is to clue us in when we're doing something out of line with our values. So if you notice you feel a surge of guilt as you reach for your fourth beer, that feeling can be useful as a helping hand to make a different choice *in the moment*. Noticing and responding when your gut says "maybe you don't want to do that" is an advantageous habit. But feeling guilt over something you did already doesn't allow you to go back in time and choose differently, it stains your current emotional landscape with negativity, and it functions exceedingly poorly at deterring future behavior.

Emotions impact the way information is interpreted, processed, stored and retrieved in the brain. The organization of data into our memory is affected by emotional context too: if you are in a positive mood right now, your brain has an easier time accessing information you learned when you were enjoying yourself. Emotional congruence dramatically increases our recollection of prior lessons. Hence, focusing on how miserable you are after a Ben & Jerry's bender is not going to be helpful when you are out with pals again, having a blast and they suggest ice cream. Likewise it's easier to recall your previous hangovers when you are curled up on the tile floor with a pounding headache, but somehow they escape your mind when there is festivity and merriment all around you and drinks are flowing.

Forgiving yourself right away if you mistakenly overeat works far better to promote leanness because it helps you feel better. Behavior change is aided by confidence and positive emotions. When we feel good, we not only believe we can do more, we actually can. We have more energy to restock the fridge with veggies, take care of ourselves and be productive with our habit practice. Don't be afraid to let yourself feel better and just keep on practicing.

To repeat: if you overeat, forgive yourself right away, and let yourself get hungry again for 30 to 60 minutes before eating. Practicing your habits gets you closer to a lean body. Practicing raking yourself over the coals doesn't.

MOVING AHEAD

As we continue into the next habits, we'll start looking at what you're eating, and show you how to get the most satisfaction per calorie with strategic and smart food choices. But these first three habits are essential to maintain. Regardless of what you eat, it is imperative that you practice feeling hunger for 30 to 60 minutes before each time you eat, stop at satisfied and stick to three or four eating occasions per day. If you need to pause here and practice these three habits until they are rock solid, feel free to do so.

Remember that while it's easiest to practice these core behaviors on "normal" days, you'll want to practice them at times that are a bit more challenging too. If you slip up and overeat at a party or on vacation, do not give up or conclude that this is impossible. Line up and give it another try—as you practice more, your skills will improve, and eventually that fiberglass windmill will be no threat at all.

Your habit tracker should now look something like this:

HABIT	1	2	3	4	5	6	7	8	9	10	11	12	13	14
Eat 3 or 4 meals without snacking														
Hunger Mastery (hunger for 30–60 minutes before eating)														
Eat just enough at each meal														

LEAN HABIT 4:
EAT MOSTLY WHOLE FOODS

At this point, we've covered the basic habits of tuning in to your body's built-in energy regulation system. Once you're consistently practicing Hunger Mastery, three or four meals is your default schedule and Eating Just Enough is second nature, you've got the best basic tools in the world for fat loss right at your fingertips—but we're nowhere near done. We haven't even talked about what's on your plate yet! Now that you are practicing hearing and heeding your body's messages about how much it needs to eat, there is still plenty more we can do to produce the calorie deficit necessary for fat loss in a comfortable manner.

WHAT TO DO

Choose foods closest to their natural state for the bulk of your meals. On your next shopping trip, try to focus on the perimeter of the store: produce, meat, dairy and refrigerated items. Can you get home without any foil bags, cardboard boxes or plastic trays?

That's not to say that all items in the center of those stores are equally processed and inherently evil—in those aisles, you'll find lentils, oatmeal and diced tomatoes, which are scarcely processed and still quite nutrient-dense choices. What we want to reduce our intake of with this habit includes items that have been highly processed (containing more than five or so ingredients is a good clue), or are hyper-palatable thanks to lots of added sugars, salt and fat. Plain frozen veggies or canned beans are not to worry about.

Think chicken breast over breaded, frozen chicken patties or whole grain oats over processed cold cereal. You don't have to go from zero to 60 all at once, just take one step closer to the farm. Instead of granola bars or chips, have fruit and nuts. Instead of a manufactured protein bar with 30 ingredients, try having some Greek yogurt for a portable source of protein.

CHOOSE FOODS CLOSEST TO THEIR NATURAL STATE FOR THE BULK OF YOUR MEALS. ON YOUR NEXT SHOPPING TRIP, TRY TO FOCUS ON THE PERIMETER OF THE STORE: PRODUCE, MEAT, DAIRY AND REFRIGERATED ITEMS. CAN YOU GET HOME WITHOUT ANY FOIL BAGS, CARDBOARD BOXES OR PLASTIC TRAYS?

You can greatly increase your nutrient intake and reduce your preservative consumption by making meals from whole foods, plus they'll help you continue toward effortless leanness by filling you up on fewer calories.

WHY IT'S WORTH IT

The appetite and satisfaction system you were born with can be fooled. Relying heavily on sugary and highly processed foods can leave you feeling hungry despite consuming thousands of calories. With this habit, we'll make sure that most of the foods you eat are unprocessed, whole foods, which will avoid short-circuiting the body's energy-balance system and keep you losing weight.

Our bodies are designed to not only survive, but thrive, on real, unprocessed foods. Whole foods are simply foods that are closest to their natural state. Like high-octane fuel in a premium sports car, whole foods nourish your body and keep you running at peak performance.

But in today's rushed world, convenience foods like quick microwaveable meals or easy-to-grab protein bars often replace whole foods in our diets. Unfortunately, what we gain in convenience comes at a cost—the more processed foods we eat, the harder it is to meet nutrient-intake guidelines. It also gets in the way of attaining leanness goals, since processed foods are higher in calorie density, which thwarts our body's natural appetite regulation system and cues us to eat more than we need.

HOW IT WORKS

The industrialized food industry has grown rapidly over the last century. While our grandparents once farmed or knew their local farmers by first name, modern Americans consume 57 percent of total energy, 52 percent of saturated fat, and 75 percent of added sugars from processed, low-nutrient sources. We also spend time browsing Pinterest and Facebook or driving to the store instead of hunting and gathering. It's no coincidence that these transitions have been accompanied by pandemic obesity.

Whole foods generally provide more nutrition than processed foods. Every step in processing strips foods of their natural structure and irreplaceable synergistic nutrients. For example, consider the difference between a fresh carrot, frozen sliced carrots and carrot cake mix. Each processing step reduces vitamin and mineral content and destroys multitudes of valuable phytochemicals.

Modern science is only beginning to elucidate the health benefits of phytochemicals, many of which provide protection against cancer, cardiovascular disease, diseases of inflammation and diabetes. Although we've identified thousands of beneficial plant compounds, scientists expect to discover hundreds more each year.

Whole foods assist in weight loss because they generally contain fewer calories per unit of weight, thanks to having a lot of water and fibrous cell walls. These structural components even decrease the percentage of calories you absorb from whole foods, because your body has to do more work to digest and assimilate nutrients when cell walls and dietary fiber are present.

The surefire way to get every last calorie from some grains of wheat? Grind them into flour, throw away the pesky germ and bran and dry them out. Take it one step further by turning this readily digested flour into a cereal with artificial colors and flavor enhancers, and you've got a recipe for maximal weight gain. You'll find greater appetite satisfaction from a cup of cooked sweet potato than you would from the same amount of sweet potato made into fries or chips.

Choosing whole foods aligns well with Eating Just Enough. Additives like sugar, salt and hard-to-pronounce chemicals dull our palates; we become accustomed to these exaggerated flavors and lose our appreciation for their healthy alternatives. These additives also impact blood sugar and brain chemistry, making it more difficult to sense our true hunger and fullness cues—and as a result, make it easier to overeat. Highly sweetened foods even produce brain activity patterns similar in ways to drugs of addiction like cocaine, morphine or heroin. Whether or not these foods qualify as "addictive" or not remains open to debate (and the definition of addiction itself is equally nebulous), but it is safe to say that they are in some ways *too tasty* for our own good if consumed frequently or in large quantities.

Whole foods are highly appetite satisfying because they take more effort and time to consume (consider peeling and eating three whole oranges or a glass of OJ for the same calories—which takes more effort and, in the end, is more satisfying?) and they release nutrients more slowly into the bloodstream. The dietary fiber contained in whole foods not only provides health benefits but also contributes to appetite satisfaction.

PUTTING THE WHOLE-FOODS HABIT INTO PRACTICE

With my coaching clients, personalizing this habit often involves a detailed discussion about particular items the client eats regularly.

While some foods are clearly whole and unprocessed (apples, eggs, almonds) and some foods clearly aren't (Lean Cuisine, Cheetos, Special K bars), there's a lot of middle ground and many shades of gray. Most clients will ask a series of questions like, "So is cheese a whole food? How about my protein powder? Can I eat jarred tomato sauce?" and so forth.

Fight the urge to divide foods into "good" and "bad" categories. You don't need a list of foods that are "okay" and "not okay," I promise. Successfully reaping the benefits of this habit simply means looking at processed foods in your diet and considering less processed alternatives. With practice, you might even find you prefer less processed versions of food you once considered "a staple."

One-hundred percent, straight-from-the-farm items won't comprise all of your meals all of the time; just try to take a step closer in areas that feel manageable to you. A great place for many weight-loss-minded people to begin is by replacing refined starch "diet foods" like rice cakes and one-hundred-calorie packs of cookies or crackers with real, satisfying foods. Another good swap is to have fruit for dessert, or real food protein instead of a bar or shake. (If you are consuming more than one protein supplement a day, it's an especially good idea to pare back a bit.) If you rely on fast food or frozen meals due to a cooking aversion, you might be surprised to find it's not much more work to make sandwiches, soup or simple meals on your own with a few ingredients. Even non-cooks can typically make eggs, a burger and salad, or a grilled-cheese sandwich and microwaved vegetables.

MOST IS BETTER THAN ALL

Stressing over "not being able" to buy canned tomatoes is counterproductive to weight loss. Likewise, if you're worrying how you'll learn to make your own yogurt, build a chicken coop or find time to bake your own bread, relax. Please notice that I specified *mostly* whole foods. Thinking that you have to eat *only* whole foods won't earn you extra credit; in fact I strongly discourage you from making that your aim! Swearing off any food completely or making a rigid rule about it isn't part of a sustainable, balanced plan. All of the habits have some flexibility, so you'll rarely see the words *always* or *never* used in my coaching books or articles. It simply wouldn't be truthful to say that you have to switch to all whole foods to get lean. That's a lie. You can get lean having some chocolate every now and then, or a slice of pizza, or a blueberry muffin. Research supports that eating mostly whole foods is a good idea for great health; you don't have to go overboard and extend that to 100 percent though.

Add "Eat mostly whole foods" to your tracker and start practicing your new habit!

HABIT	1	2	3	4	5	6	7	8	9	10	11	12	13	14
Eat 3 or 4 meals without snacking														
Hunger Mastery (hunger for 30–60 minutes before eating)														
Eat just enough at each meal														
Eat mostly (or all) whole foods														

LEAN HABIT 5:

EAT VEGETABLES, AND LOTS OF THEM

WHAT TO DO

Aim to eat two to three cups of vegetables with each meal. For most people that means you'll tally up six to nine cups of vegetables per day. If it's easier to think in terms of weight, I recommend getting 300 grams or more of veggies at every meal, which is about 10 ounces. But you can certainly go above that. Generally, there's no amount of vegetables that will harm you from a health standpoint; the only things that you may experience with extreme vegetable overload are an orange color to your skin or some digestive discomfort. The orange skin color, known as carotenoderma, results from a high intake of carotenoids, and is sometimes seen in people who eat several servings of carrots and yams every day. It's harmless; it never happens to most people even if you do eat these foods daily, and it reverses if you back off the carrots.

If you develop gastrointestinal discomfort, such as gas pains or bloating, while increasing your vegetable intake, make sure to cook your vegetables thoroughly (especially ones in the cabbage family like broccoli, cauliflower and brussels sprouts) and avoid any that specifically upset your belly. With hundreds of vegetables to choose from, it's not a big problem to discover that some digest more easily for you than others. There are plenty left to choose from! Over-the-counter products like Beano can help reduce gas if taken with meals, too. If you have a condition like irritable bowel or colitis, and many types of vegetables give you trouble, a registered dietitian can help you plan meals and find ways to get your veggies in without upsetting your stomach.

Salads and stir-fries are just the beginning. You can enjoy your vegetables roasted, grilled, steamed, sautéed, pureed or simmered into soups and stews. You can bake them, cook them into omelets, layer them into casseroles or crunch on them raw; just eat them.

Remember that eating well does not have to be boring. Look for recipes online and aim for vegetables in a variety of types and colors.

See the list below for ideas:

- Acorn Squash
- Arugula
- Artichokes
- Asparagus
- Bean Sprouts
- Beets
- Bell Peppers
- Bok Choy
- Broccoli
- Brussels Sprouts
- Butternut Squash
- Cabbage
- Carrots
- Cauliflower
- Celery
- Collard Greens
- Cucumber

- Eggplant
- Endive
- Fennel
- Green Beans
- Jalapeños
- Jicama
- Kale
- Kohlrabi
- Leek
- Lettuce
- Mustard Greens
- Okra
- Onion
- Parsnip
- Peppers
- Pumpkin
- Radicchio

- Radish
- Rutabaga
- Snow Peas
- Spaghetti Squash
- Spinach
- Sugar Snap Peas
- Swiss Chard
- Tomato
- Turnip
- Turnip Greens
- Watercress
- Wax Beans
- Yellow Summer Squash
- Yellow Tomatoes
- Zucchini

Don't panic if you're not currently eating many vegetables. Just start wherever you are. If you eat only one or two cups of vegetables a day, try to get to three cups a day for a while before increasing more.

WHY IT'S WORTH IT

While this book is focused on fat loss, consider how high vegetable intake has been shown to reduce the risk of cancer, cardiovascular disease, coronary heart disease, stroke, diabetes and obesity. Having a longer, healthier life seems worth mentioning at least once as its own benefit—fat loss isn't all there is to good nutrition. Sure, I want to be rocking a bikini at the beach, but more importantly, I want to still be around to enjoy the beach in another 50 years.

Since we're talking about shedding fat, let's focus on how eating lots of veggies helps you get leaner. To drop fat without getting too uncomfortable, you want appetite satiety without excess calories at every meal. Enter vegetables.

HOW IT WORKS

Sure vegetables happen to be packed with health-promoting phytochemicals, vitamins, minerals and fiber, but their fat-loss power lies in what they are relatively lacking in: calories. Vegetables are the least calorie-dense food group. Period.

Vegetables contain lots of water, plus indigestible carbohydrates known as dietary fiber, which add volume to your plate and help you achieve fullness for very few calories. By increasing the amount of real estate on your dinner plate allotted to veggies, you will naturally crowd out higher-calorie foods. If you start your meal with a big salad and enjoy a generous portion of roasted broccoli or zucchini, it's not hard to imagine being satisfied with smaller portions of meat and starch, the more calorie-concentrated items.

A 2013 study showed that reducing the energy density of entrees by 20 percent with fruits and vegetables reduced subjects' consumption by 308 calories over the course of the day—even when allowed to eat freely. So without thinking about it, you could comfortably reduce calorie intake and lose weight, just by adding more vegetables to your meals.

Speaking of comfort, research also shows that a low-energy-density diet is much more comfortable to sustain than a high-energy-dense diet of the same calories. If the foundation of your diet is calorie-dense foods like granola, cheese, crackers and nuts, for a given amount of calories, your food volume is very small. The stretch receptors in your stomach aren't as stimulated, and it's incredibly easy to eat more calories than you need.

I like comfort. I'm interested in making getting lean as comfortable as possible for you too. A 2010 research study found that women consuming 1,500 calories a day from meals high in fruits and vegetables reported significantly less hunger than women consuming the same amount of calories but with less emphasis on produce. Both groups lost similar amounts of weight, but the vegetable-heavy group ate more than twice the volume of food! If I can eat four pounds of food a day and my neighbor only eats two pounds, and we both lose the same amount of weight, I'd definitely feel like the lucky one (and she might be blaming her metabolism). But it's not luck, it's just going heavy on the plants!

Larger population-based studies have found the same thing: Americans who eat the most fruits and vegetables have the lowest prevalence of obesity. They have a lower energy intake, yet they consume 300 to 400 grams more food each day than those who eat less fruits and vegetables. That's almost a pound more food.

Want even more reasons to aim for a high vegetable intake beyond filling you up and slimming you down?

Increased vegetable consumption has been shown to favorably affect the expression of genes that regulate energy metabolism while controlling inflammation and oxidative stress. This may help improve glucose tolerance and fuel utilization and the adaptive response to exercise, all of which are beneficial for those seeking to be their physical best.

WHAT ABOUT FRUIT?

Like vegetables, fruit is also relatively low in calorie density, and can be a naturally sweet treat that packs many of the same nutrients. While I don't recommend replacing vegetables with fruit, you can certainly gain additional benefits from adding one or two pieces of fruit to your day's meals, especially if they replace desserts or processed foods. If you struggle with getting two cups of vegetables into breakfast, try one cup of vegetables and one cup of fruit instead.

TIP: YOU'RE GOING TO HAVE TO BUY MORE PRODUCE

If you purchase the same amount of vegetables you always have but double your intake, you're going to run out a lot sooner, you vegetable-chomping superstar. So before mindlessly getting the same-old, same-old at the grocery store, remember that you're upgrading your vegetable-intake habits, so your shopping cart needs to match. Pick up extra servings of your usual veggies, and try a new variety or two if you like.

If you're concerned because you already end up throwing away vegetables and don't want to simply have more produce go to waste, do this experiment: keep them on the top shelf of your refrigerator, not in the drawers at the bottom where they are easily forgotten. Yes, even though they may be labeled for fruits and veggies, the "crisper" drawers aren't the best spot to put your veggies unless you want to forget about them and throw them out after they've gone slimy. The reduced airflow of the drawers is intended to keep vegetables from drying out or wilting, but it's just as effective to keep them in the clear produce bags they came in. Poke a hole in the bag (a thumb works) and leave them on the upper shelves of the fridge, high up where you will not miss them or forget you have them. As for those drawers, use one for raw meat to keep it separate from other foods in case of leaks, and fill the other with yogurts, cheese or other items with a longer shelf life, like onions, apples and turnips.

FAQ: WHAT VEGGIES GO WELL WITH BREAKFAST?

People often have an easier time loading up on vegetables at lunch and dinner, but breakfast can be tricky. Eggs go fabulously with vegetables, so you can toss peppers, mushrooms and onions into your omelet or scramble. If you need a make-ahead meal, a quiche or frittata can also be a place to add spinach, kale, onions or eggplant. Greens like spinach and kale blend beautifully into shakes and smoothies. Canned pumpkin is a tasty addition to oatmeal, hot cereal, pancakes or yogurt. For a simple solution, raw sliced tomato is an easy no-cook side dish, or grab a handful of grape tomatoes.

Time to update your tracker and get started with practicing. You might phrase this habit as "Eat at least six cups of vegetables" or "Eat two to three cups of vegetables with every meal." Remember, you can scale this habit; if jumping up to two to three cups per meal is too large of a change, you can set an interim goal as you work your way up. You tracker should now look like this:

HABIT	1	2	3	4	5	6	7	8	9	10	11	12	13	14
Eat 3 or 4 meals without snacking														
Hunger Mastery (hunger for 30–60 minutes before eating)														
Eat just enough at each meal														
Eat mostly (or all) whole foods														
Eat at least 6 cups of vegetables														

LEAN HABIT 6:
MINIMIZE LIQUID CALORIES

As mentioned in the "Appetite Satisfaction" section of the introduction, the physical attributes of your food choices affect how satisfying they are. Foods that have more volume and are solid (as opposed to liquid) give you more appetite satisfaction and fullness than low-volume or liquid sources of calories.

Guess what? You're already practicing some habits that capitalize on this! Eating whole foods and loading up on vegetables have already helped to steer you towards meals that include fiber-filled and high-volume items. They'll stay in your stomach longer, activate those stretch receptors and send more fullness signals to your brain than low-volume meals made from processed foods. Next, we're going to focus specifically on liquid calories, which may be the least satisfying and most weight-gain promoting of all calories you consume.

WHAT TO DO

Pay attention to the liquid calories you consume on a daily basis. If you want to dive right in and go for optimal, start right now by drinking nothing but water or other calorie-free drinks. If that's a bit too daunting of a change, start by reducing portions of the calorie-containing drinks you enjoy. You can also set a goal for yourself to have only a set number of calorie-containing drinks per week, and reduce it as you get comfortable. It can be a pleasant change to discover new beverages to replace the old ones, so check out sparkling water, make your own unsweetened iced tea or investigate a new exotic hot tea. Make it your goal to eventually consume as close to zero calories from beverages as possible.

If protein shakes and smoothies are part of your diet, these also are worth attention to. It's easy to throw 300 to 500 calories of fruit, protein powder, and other tasty ingredients into a blender, whip them into a delicious concoction and drink it down easily. While not fully liquid, smoothies and shakes are much closer to liquid than solid foods, and they also empty from the stomach faster and leave you feeling hunger sooner than a calorie-equivalent meal of solid food would. If you want to take an extra step toward being satisfied on fewer calories, consider replacing some or all of the shakes/smoothies in your diet with solid-food meals. If the convenience of a smoothie or protein shake is something you just can't live without, keep it to one per day or only on days when your schedule really necessitates it.

WHY IT'S WORTH IT

It's no coincidence that the expanding waistlines of our population coincide with our increasing liquid-calorie consumption. Liquid calories in the form of soda, sweet tea, fruit juices, milk, fruit smoothies, sports drinks, energy drinks, coffee drinks, beer and wine increase calorie intake without satisfying your appetite. Eliminating liquid calories from your diet helps promote weight loss and better nutrition. The payoffs don't end with a slimmer body, either. Consumption of sugar-sweetened beverages not only raises your risk for becoming obese, it also increases your odds of developing type 2 diabetes and cardiovascular disease.

Like a co-worker that does not pull their weight, it is time to give the boot to these empty calories that don't earn their keep.

HOW IT WORKS

"Wow, that Big Gulp was so satisfying!" said no one, ever. There are 400 calories in just one 32-ounce soda, or about 20 percent of the amount an active adult needs in a whole day. And it won't even put a dent in your hunger at mealtime.

Perhaps you wouldn't ever think of having a Big Gulp, but many health-conscious adults still consume fruit juice and milk, which are more nutritious than soda but still provide hundreds of calories with little effect on diminishing appetite. For example, a 16-ounce glass of orange juice in the morning and a 16-ounce nonfat latte (no whipped cream or sugar) is 350 calories. For the same calories, you could eat an entire plate of food: a quarter pound of roasted chicken and a pile of roasted veggies with olive oil. Which of these do you think would leave you more satisfied—a couple of drinks or the plate of food?

During digestion, whole foods require both time and energy to be broken down. This process naturally slows the rate at which nutrients enter the bloodstream, resulting in stabilized blood sugar and prolonged stomach fullness. Liquids, on the other hand, digest quickly and produce a quick rise and steep decline in blood sugar, predisposing the consumer to increased cravings, inflammation, beta cell dysfunction and abdominal fat storage. Liquid calories also fool our appetite control system because they don't register with the brain and produce the normal responses (such as decreased appetite) that occur when we eat a meal of solid food.

CLINICAL TRIAL DATA SHOW THAT REDUCING LIQUID CALORIES RESULTS IN MORE FAT AND WEIGHT LOSS THAN REDUCING AN IDENTICAL NUMBER OF SOLID-FOOD CALORIES. IN OTHER WORDS, PARING OUT 100 CALORIES FROM YOUR BEVERAGES CAN BE A BIGGER STEP TOWARDSWEIGHT LOSS THAN EATING 100 CALORIES LESS FOOD.

Drinking only calorie-free beverages, such as water or unsweetened iced tea, has been shown to be an effective strategy for losing weight, even when the food you eat stays the same. In fact, clinical trial data show that reducing liquid calories results in more fat and weight loss than reducing an identical number of solid-food calories. In other words, paring out 100 calories from your beverages can be a bigger step toward weight loss than eating 100 calories less food.

Results of a 2012 clinical trial published in *The American Journal of Clinical Nutrition* found that replacement of caloric beverages with non-caloric beverages as a weight-loss strategy resulted in average weight losses of 2 to 2.5 percent over six months. If you weigh 180 pounds, that means you could lose four-and-a-half pounds just from choosing only calorie-free beverages, even if you ate exactly the same things.

Cutting back on liquid calories isn't just good for adults, but for children too. Swapping just a single eight-ounce sugar-sweetened beverage for a calorie-free one has been shown to be effective in reducing fat gain and keeping children from developing obesity.

Don't underestimate the power of small changes, made consistently.

"NOT MY COFFEE, ANYTHING BUT THAT!"

For many people, the daily coffee ritual is nothing short of sacred. However, it can also be a huge source of hidden calories you may not think about, depending on how much milk, cream or sugar you use. If you have one cup a day and use a small amount of milk or cream and little or no caloric sweeteners, your coffee habit is probably not a significant contributor to any excess weight that you carry. However, if you drink several cups a day, and pour in milk or cream from a bottle without thinking, even before you add sugar you could be swigging hundreds of calories. Start adding flavored syrups, sugar or honey, and a plain coffee can be hundreds of calories that provide practically zero satisfaction.

The best way to reduce the calories in your coffee is to start measuring the milk or cream and sugar you add, and decrease the quantity gradually. You can also reduce calories by switching to lower-calorie add-ins like calorie-free sweeteners, almond milk or lower-fat milk instead of cream. Or, if you prefer, you can simply drink less coffee. Going from four cups a day to two cuts calories in half, even if you are unwilling to budge on what you add to your cup of joe. Find the way that's most comfortable for you to reduce liquid calories, and start practicing.

I'd like to tell you about my client Catie. Catie was a nurse in the labor and delivery unit of a busy Colorado hospital, and she often had to work 12-hour shifts that went into the wee hours of the morning. In the first few weeks of coaching, she lost weight while learning to feel hunger before eating and paring out snacking. But then her weight loss just stopped. We talked about where extra calories in her diet might be coming from. She confirmed that she was eating three meals a day, successfully avoiding the pervasive junk foods available in the hospital unit, limiting her portions to just enough to be satisfied and feeling hunger for 30 to 60 minutes prior to eating. She was understandably frustrated and upset that despite all her hard work, her weight stayed stuck after the first few pounds. I asked her to log everything she ate and drank for three days with as much detail as possible, knowing together we would find something to break this plateau. I just didn't want her to give up before we found it!

I noticed on her log that in addition to her healthy meals, Catie was drinking a lot of coffee. She hadn't even written how many cups, but instead wrote "(Coffee)" in the blanks between meals. And on nights she worked, she was having coffee between every meal it seemed. She explained to me it's practically part of the job. Bringing babies into the world, unfortunately, is an unpredictable business, and if she was caring for a patient in labor she might not get to take a break long enough to eat a meal. Swigging coffee helped her stay awake, and not be as bothered by the hunger if she didn't get to eat for a while. And when it was slow, she and the other nurses would drink coffee and talk to pass the time. She figured since she didn't add sugar to her coffee that it wouldn't be a big source of calories. But since she was having four to six cups a day, I suspected the half and half might be adding up, so I asked her to measure it.

Three days and *59 tablespoons* of half and half later, we knew what we were dealing with. In three 12-hour shifts, Catie consumed almost 1,200 calories in half and half! Without even knowing it, she had taken in as many calories as if she'd eaten a whole pint of ice cream. When I told her that, she laughed and said, "Dang! I wish I had had the ice cream!"

We talked about switching to a lower-calorie alternative to add to her coffee instead of creamer, and I assured her that once she got used to it, a less calorie-laden whitener for her coffee would probably taste fine. Catie tried out regular milk, soy milk, almond milk (after which she wrote me a *very* unhappy e-mail) and coconut creamers. While most of my clients have not had much trouble switching to these other creamers to save calories, Catie really hated them all. So, she decided that she would keep drinking her coffee the way she liked it, with half and half, but cut back to just one cup per shift, and use premeasured creamers from the cafeteria so the portion didn't creep up. Three tablespoons of creamer in one cup of coffee cut her added liquid calories down to 60 a day, instead of the nearly 400 she had been drinking previously. And with the reduction in liquid calories, Catie's weight started ticking downward again at a reliable pound a week.

I think Catie's story has several great lessons in it. First, beverage calories add up fast. Second, you can do lots of things "right," but one source of hidden calories can keep you from losing weight. Third, even if you can't find a lower-calorie alternative for something you like, you can just decrease your portion size and have the original. Fourth, Catie didn't have to get to zero liquid calories or cut out all her coffee to have weight-loss success, and she ended up losing 36 pounds during the time we worked together.

Time to update your habit tracker again to record your practice with trimming liquid calories.

HABIT	1	2	3	4	5	6	7	8	9	10	11	12	13	14
Eat 3 or 4 meals without snacking														
Hunger Mastery (hunger for 30–60 minutes before eating)														
Eat just enough at each meal														
Eat mostly (or all) whole foods														
Eat at least 6 cups of vegetables														
Reduce or eliminate liquid calories														

LEAN HABIT 7:
BOOST SATIETY WITH PROTEIN

WHAT TO DO

Want to boost your satiety? Keep energy stable?

Include a protein-rich food with each meal, such as eggs, egg whites, seafood, meat, poultry, soy products, cottage cheese or Greek yogurt. That means that a breakfast of fruit and cereal probably isn't going to cut it, nor will a "dinner" of canned tomato soup and some rice. While protein powders can be used in a pinch, whole food sources are best. Aiming for a palm-sized amount of cooked meat (about four ounces) works beautifully as an easy portion guide, or a fist-size serving of eggs, cottage cheese or Greek yogurt (about one cup).

If you prefer to think in terms of numbers, I recommend starting with 30 to 40 grams of protein at each of your three or four meals. The aforementioned four ounces of cooked meat will be 32 grams and the rest of the food you eat will boost the number some more. Without getting embroiled in detailed logging, this is also a foolproof way for most people to get close to the 30 percent of calories from protein backed up by extensive research. If you are having three meals a day, shoot for closer to 40 grams at each, and if you include a fourth feeding, aim for closer to 30 grams per meal.

If your calorie needs are unusually high or low you can adjust these numbers a bit, but they are suitable for you if your calorie intake falls between 1,200 and 2,000 calories a day, which is a suitable weight-loss range for most adults. Consuming fewer than 1,200 calories is not something I recommend due to the challenges it creates regarding nutrient adequacy, and if you require above 2,000 calories a day, you'll want to eat a bit more protein. It's not any problem to have extra protein, so don't worry if your intake naturally falls above my general guidelines. As long as you are seeing results, the extra calories aren't a problem.

As always, you'll want to also keep practicing Eating Just Enough, so don't leave all your protein for last at mealtime; you don't want to be faced with deciding to eat past satiety just to get your protein in. If you find yourself in that scenario on a regular basis, try eating the protein-rich foods first at meals, and aiming for the lower end of the 30- to 40-gram range. It only takes three ounces of cooked chicken to get 25 grams of protein, so it's not a ton of food. Remember that you'll also be getting a few grams of protein from the vegetables you eat, and if you add beans, dairy or nuts to your meal, protein grams can add up quickly and easily.

In my experience, most clients who are learning this habit for the first time are consuming too little protein at breakfast (10 to 20 grams), and many are consuming excessively large portions when they eat meat or poultry (a large chicken breast can be 50 grams of protein). They feel better and have an easier time losing weight when they even it out into 30 to 40 total grams of protein consistently at every meal.

To look up the amount of protein in foods, try NutritionData.com and, of course, read labels. Here is a list of some commonly consumed protein-rich foods, so you can get an idea of how much your typical meals add up to. If you have a kitchen scale, I suggest using it for a few days to get an idea of how much protein you dish up in your normal portions of meat.

Dairy

- 1 cup milk = 8 grams protein
- ½ cup cottage cheese = 14 grams
- 1 ounce hard cheese = 7 to 8 grams (usually, there's some variance)
- 1 ounce soft cheese (like goat cheese) = 4 to 5 grams (usually, some variance)
- ¾ cup Greek yogurt = 18 to 21 grams

Meats (Raw)

- 4 ounces lean ground turkey = 22 grams
- 4 ounces chicken breast = 24 grams
- 4 ounces extra lean ground beef = 23 grams
- 4 ounces lean ground beef = 22 grams
- 4 ounces raw shrimp = 15 grams
- 4 ounces raw fish = 20 grams

Meats (Cooked)

- Most lean meats (skinless poultry, extra lean beef, pork tenderloin) = 8 grams per cooked ounce
- Fattier meats = 7 grams per cooked ounce
- Shrimp = 6 grams per cooked ounce
- Fish = 8 grams per cooked ounce

Eggs

- 1 large egg = 6 grams
- ¼ cup liquid egg whites = 6 grams
- 1 egg white (from a shell egg) = 4 grams

Legumes

- ½ cup garbanzo beans = 6 grams
- ½ cup black beans = 7 grams
- ½ cup edamame (edible parts) = 8 grams (that's 1⅓ cups unshelled beans)
- 4 ounces tempeh = 20 grams

Like any other food, too much protein will simply lead to taking in too many calories, so if you find you're getting above 40 grams regularly at meals and your weight loss is slow in coming, you would probably benefit from paring back. I've had clients check their normal portions of steak or chicken on a scale and find out they typically have 10 ounces of cooked meat at dinner. That's more than twice the appropriate amount even an active man needs. For most people, a portion of cooked meat that is about four ounces is plenty for a meal. If you have three and a half or five ounces, it's nothing to worry about; oversized portions simply may slow your weight loss by providing excess calories. Since meat and seafood lose water when you cook them, remember that the raw weight will be higher then the cooked weight. To get 4 ounces of cooked chicken, you'll need to start with 5–6 ounces raw.

WHY IT'S WORTH IT

Most people eat more than enough protein to maintain optimal health. True protein deficiency in developed nations is virtually absent. However, if you're interested in doing more than preventing deficiency and are seeking optimal health and a lean body composition, going above the minimal requirement provides a host of benefits. The average North American diet provides 17 percent of calories from protein, but consuming extra protein above that has been shown to curb appetite and assist in building and maintaining muscle and preventing the loss of lean tissue when losing fat. In short, it makes getting lean easier.

HOW IT WORKS

Including a substantial amount of protein with a meal helps turn on the appetite-satisfaction signals in your gut. Research subjects given higher-protein meals report greater fullness and decreased hunger than those on normal protein intakes who are taking in the same calories. This is because protein triggers a greater release of gut hormones CCK, PYY and GLP-1 compared to eating the same amount of calories from carbohydrates or fat. Recall that these hormones are part of the signals converging at the hypothalamus to give you the feeling of being full.

While scientific evidence consistently supports that adding protein to your diet helps you take in fewer calories, it remains unclear whether boosting protein helps boost energy output in a meaningful way. Some studies have shown that higher protein intakes result in 2 to 3 percent higher resting metabolic rate, the thermic effect of food, or total daily energy expenditure. However, other studies have found zero change in energy expenditure in similar conditions. So it's not certain if adding extra protein provides a small increase in energy expenditure, but it might.

The power of protein to suppress appetite appears to be dose-dependent, which means that more protein (as a percentage of total calories) produces greater appetite satisfaction. Some evidence also indicates that people who consume more protein have lower levels of abdominal fat. Compared to a normal protein diet of 18 percent of calories from protein, people eating 30 percent of calories from protein have greater appetite satisfaction, less hunger and better fat-burning ability, as evidenced by lower respiratory quotient; and when allowed to eat freely they naturally eat fewer calories.

When someone is deliberately eating at a caloric deficit to lose weight, getting 30 percent of total calories from protein has even more benefits. The additional protein in the diet preserves more muscle mass compared to a normal protein (18 percent) diet, ensuring that a higher percentage of pounds lost come from fat. Weight-loss diets with 30 percent of calories from protein also significantly improve perceptions of fullness and pleasure, both of which greatly increase your chances of adhering to the diet for a length of time and reaching your goal weight.

Higher protein intake also correlates with retaining muscle mass as we age, regardless of physical activity levels. Keeping muscle tissue not only helps people look strong and shapely, it allows them to preserve their metabolic rate and prevent the gradual weight gain associated with aging.

More protein isn't necessarily better, however. The preponderance of studies showing the benefits of higher protein intakes have utilized levels at or about 30 percent of total calories. This doesn't mean that 40 or 50 percent of calories from protein would be more advantageous in any way. At some point, adding extra protein-rich food to the diet simply becomes counterproductive for fat loss as it entails intake of unneeded calories, which can be turned into body fat. Besides, for optimal health, well-being and athletic performance, a person needs to leave room in the diet for adequate carbohydrates and fats as well.

Time to update your tracker, and start off two weeks practicing your new habit.

HABIT	1	2	3	4	5	6	7	8	9	10	11	12	13	14
Eat 3 or 4 meals without snacking														
Hunger Mastery (hunger for 30–60 minutes before eating)														
Eat just enough at each meal														
Eat mostly (or all) whole foods														
Eat at least 6 cups of vegetables														
Reduce or eliminate liquid calories														
30–40 grams of protein at each meal														

LEAN HABIT 8:
EAT THE RIGHT AMOUNT OF FAT

WHAT TO DO

"We don't want high fat or low fat, we want <u>moderate fat</u>."

I recommend starting by aiming for about 15 grams of fat with each meal. They might just be the most satisfying calories you eat, especially if you don't like obsessing over how hungry you are between meals. Eating fewer than 15 grams of fat at a meal is something I recommend only if for some reason you want to be hungry again soon, such as if you end up eating two meals relatively close together and you want to be hungry for the second meal. For maximum satisfaction, approximately 15 grams usually is the lowest amount needed to keep you satisfied if you expect to not eat again for five or six hours. Please do not stress if you are a couple grams over or under, I said *about* 15 grams. These are not atomic weapons, they are grams of oil; a few each way is *fine*.

The easiest no-fuss way to hit your moderate-fat target is to get familiar with what foods are sources of fat and *approximate* how much you're having. You might find that your usual breakfast of hard-boiled egg whites, tomatoes and toast with a teaspoon of butter only comes to five grams of fat, so you'll want to add some more fat by cooking with olive oil, adding a whole egg or garnishing it with some avocado or cheese. Or, you might start eyeballing the fat content in your steak dinner and realize that your side salad alone has 25 grams of fat from a tablespoon of olive oil and ounce of shredded cheese, so before you've touched the steak or oiled vegetables in front of you, you've gone beyond your fat needs.

If you find you are consuming much less than this amount, easy ways to add 5 grams of fat are to add one additional teaspoon of oil or butter, one ounce of avocado or a half-ounce of cheese to your meal. I *never* have a hard time eating a tablespoon of nut butter for an extra 8 grams of fat if my meal is on the low side, and many of my clients enjoy it too. (Have you been avoiding peanut butter because of the fat in it? Well go get some! Life's too short to avoid delicious things, and in the right amounts they can help you get leaner.)

If you find you're having far more fat than 15 or 20 grams at a meal, try to bring the fat down by getting in the habit of choosing just one or two fat sources at each meal (for instance, choosing cheese *or* nuts *or* dressing for your salad instead of all three). Don't forget that meat, chicken, cheese and fish all contain some fat too, so you will be getting some grams of fat in your protein source already and may not need to add much more.

I cannot emphasize enough that for this to become a maintainable habit, it's not about logging fat grams or counting fractions of a gram of fat from the beans in your chili. The goal is to get out of the habit of making meals with too little fat, and to avoid adding hundreds of extra calories by using too much of it. Instead, you'll form the habit of enjoying some fat with each meal in a moderate portion.

Can you go above 15 grams of fat per meal? Of course. It's a guideline for the lowest effective amount. But don't go too crazy on the coconut oil yet. High-fat diets (more than 40 percent of calories from fat) actually decrease the sensitivity of the hypothalamus to leptin and other hormones involved in appetite regulation. The reward value of high-fat foods also decreases if fat intake is too high. After even a short time consuming a high-fat diet, our brain releases less dopamine in response to eating, making food less pleasurable and satisfying. Evidence from human and animal studies supports that this weakened food-reward circuitry may underlie behavior to seek more and more food and develop obesity. So keep it moderate.

Obviously, more fat in your meal means more calories. You want enough fat to ensure you stay satisfied until 30 to 60 minutes before you eat again, but it's just adding calories above that point. If your weight loss is progressing fine, then you aren't taking in too many calories, so don't sweat it. But if your weight is not coming down, some quick math to see if you're habitually having high-fat meals might be the troubleshoot you need. To get weight loss going, your calorie intake needs to be lower, and reducing extra fat is often the easiest place to trim calories. If you are taking in more than 40 percent of calories from fat, weight loss is a bit tougher. So if you eat an average of 1,800 calories a day, 80 grams would be the maximum amount I'd recommend.

As for the types of fat you should include, there is little evidence that specific types of fat are any more or less appetite satisfying or "fattening." But there are dramatic health benefits to consuming monounsaturated fats (olives, olive oil, avocado) and omega-3 polyunsaturates (fish, seafood, flaxseed, chia seed). I encourage my clients to include monounsaturated and omega-3 fats every day, and choose additional fats from a variety of whole-food fat sources like nuts, seeds, meats, coconut and dairy foods to their liking. One kind of fat that is best avoided is trans fat, found in partially hydrogenated oils, an ingredient in many processed foods.

WHY 15-ISH GRAMS, ANYWAY?

I didn't pull these numbers out of thin air; they are based on what nutrition research indicates is a beneficial level of fat for health and leanness: close to 30 percent of total calories. Choosing 15 grams of fat at each meal and eating three or four meals works out to be close enough to the optimal zone of 30 percent of calorie intake for people eating 1,350 to 1,800 calories a day (which encompasses the needs of most adults losing weight, and interestingly, is the calorie range where people using the Lean Habits system tend to unknowingly gravitate).

WHY IT'S WORTH IT

If you've been struggling with your weight for years, you may have gotten into the habit of avoiding fat and choosing low-fat foods and cooking methods to save calories. Or, like many people, you may be taking in too much fat, because you love the taste of cheese, French fries or creamy sauces. Neither is optimal for getting and staying lean. Whether you consume too little or too much fat right now, practicing the habit of building meals with a moderate amount of fat has benefits in helping you control your appetite, manage your calorie intake, keep your body metabolically flexible and, ultimately, have an easier time losing weight.

High fat diets (defined as greater than 40 percent of calories from fat) typically lead to high calorie intakes and becoming or staying overweight. In a laboratory setting, covertly changing the fat content of people's diets results in them consuming 15 percent more calories on a diet that provides 45 to 50 percent of calories as fat, compared to a moderate fat diet providing 30 to 35 percent of calories as fat. Over a two-week period, this was enough to cause a statistically significant weight gain. Because fat is very calorie dense (nine calories per gram, more than twice the calorie content of protein or carbohydrate), overshooting your calorie needs with cheese or peanut butter is easy to do without noticing a change in food volume. Because high-fat foods are also highly palatable (Cheese! Peanut butter! Two of my favorites, for the record), it's easy to overshoot one's calorie needs when enjoying higher-fat foods just because they taste so good. Obviously that doesn't aid weight loss. A high-fat diet paired with energy excess also decreases insulin sensitivity and impairs metabolic flexibility and glucose handling. The stage is then set for the development of chronic inflammation, worsening many existing health conditions and predisposing a person to developing others.

Research has implicated high fat intake as a causative factor in the development of leptin resistance, a state in which the brain is rendered handicapped to appropriately sense fuel abundance in the body. Leptin resistance favors continual weight gain over time, so it's not something you want. Exposure to a diet with greater than 40 percent of calories from fat has been shown to weaken the body's sensitivity to other hormones too, such as CCK and GLP-1, both of which are critical to feeling satisfied after a meal. In other words, consuming a high-fat diet on a regular basis leaves you more inflamed, favors taking in more calories and gaining weight, and damages the mechanisms your body uses to feel satisfied on the appropriate amount of food. Yikes.

The fat we eat impacts more than energy-balance circuits in the brain. It's involved in reward circuits and pleasure sensing as well! Functional MRI studies have shown that when we eat fat-containing foods, it activates the lateral hypothalamus, amygdala, insula and anterior cingulate cortex areas of the brain which light up when you do something rewarding (not just getting enough calories). At moderate fat intakes this isn't a problem, but chronic high-dietary fat intake decreases dopamine signaling in the brain, essentially muting the reward circuits. Experts in neurochemistry believe that this dulling of the reward value of food leaves a person chasing the high, so to speak, consuming greater quantities of food overall and favoring selection of more hyperpalatable foods packed with sugar, salt and more fat over their less-processed alternatives.

So high-fat diets obviously aren't the cat's meow, but don't rush to throw out your butter or pour the olive oil down the drain! Low-fat diets create problems all their own. In the 1980s and 1990s, low-fat diets were widely recommended by doctors, dietitians and government health bodies, as it was believed they not only helped to control weight but also assisted with cardiovascular disease prevention. (It turned out that they weren't beneficial for either.)

In the 1990s I consumed my body weight annually in fat-free Rold Gold pretzels and Snackwell's cookies. I couldn't figure out why I was hungry all the time. And millions of other people were doing the exact same thing I was. Encouraged by the promise of low-fat weight loss, North Americans slashed fat grams, buying low-fat margarines, spooning up nonfat yogurt to go with their egg-white omelets and crunching on fat-free potato chips in front of the television. And they only got heavier. How did that happen? Because as dietary fat went *down*, total calories consumed went *up*.

In the last 15 years, research studies have revealed some of the pitfalls of low-fat dieting. Low-fat diets (less than 25 percent calories from fat) fall short on appetite satisfaction, making them unfavorable for sustaining leanness; as we know, you won't sustain anything forever if you aren't getting satisfied. Recent research supports that a more moderate fat intake (around 30 percent) is superior for long-term weight loss because this level offers better hunger suppression, encourages greater food variety and provides greater enjoyment. Furthermore, eating a diet with a moderate amount of fat is more effective than a low-fat diet for improving blood lipids and cardiovascular disease risk. At this moderate level, the consumer can avoid the undesired effects seen when fat climbs above 40 percent of daily calorie intake.

Most low-fat-diet studies were not carried out for long periods of time. Weight-loss studies consistently show that people can (and will) do just about anything for one to six months and lose weight. Low-fat diets, low-carbohydrate diets and liquid diets … they all work in the short term. The true test is how well people can stick to the methods that helped them lose weight to avoid regain year after year.

In the long term, research supports that people on *moderate*-fat diets lose more weight and body fat than fat avoiders; they also stick to their diet longer without quitting than those who use a low-fat approach. In a clinical trial comparing the long-term compliance and efficacy of low-fat and moderate-fat diets, both performed equally well for the first six months. But then it got interesting. The low-fat group had dramatically higher dropout rates as the months went by, and by the end of the 18-month study, the low-fat diet group had regained all the pounds they lost initially, and ended up weighing in at above their starting weight. The moderate-fat group had fewer dropouts and maintained their weight losses through the 18-month mark.

IN THE LONG TERM, RESEARCH SUPPORTS THAT PEOPLE ON *MODERATE*-FAT DIETS LOSE MORE WEIGHT AND BODY FAT THAN FAT AVOIDERS; THEY ALSO STICK TO THEIR DIET LONGER WITHOUT QUITTING THAN THOSE WHO USE A LOW-FAT APPROACH.

Similar findings were reported in a study published in the *New England Journal of Medicine*. Compared to a moderate-fat Mediterranean diet, and a high-fat, low-carbohydrate diet, the low-fat diet produced less weight loss, greater weight rebound and lower diet compliance over a two-year study in obese adults. The low-fat diet also performed the *worst* of the three diets in improving blood cholesterol levels and C-reactive protein. Diabetic participants in the low-fat diet group had higher fasting blood glucose values at the end of the study (indicating their blood sugar control had worsened), while both of the other groups saw improvements in glucose tolerance.

Following up with the same subjects four years later provided an interesting look at what happens in the years after someone goes on a diet. Subjects on the low-fat diet lost the least weight during the study and regained it all during the follow-up period, achieving no significant weight loss at the end of six years. All that work for nothing. The people randomized to follow a high-fat but low-carb diet lost weight fast during the trial but regained most of it back during the follow-up period. The people on the moderate-fat Mediterranean diet fared the best in the long run; they lost almost as much weight as those on the low-carb, high-fat diet during the study, but while the other two groups packed the pounds back on, the moderate-fat dieters kept most of their weight off, even four years after the study ended.

This is consistent with what I see in my clients all the time. High-fat diets are usually high-calorie diets, and lead to people gaining unwanted weight. When it comes to weight loss, cutting fat too low, or cutting back on carbs to try to lose weight with a high-fat Paleo or low-carb diet, only works in the short term. Either extreme leaves a person too hungry or deprived, and they gain the weight back. I really don't want that to happen to you. It's worth it to learn how to eat a moderate-fat diet.

HOW IT WORKS

Dietary fat helps you reach fullness when eating. Consuming fat with a meal triggers the release of satiety hormones like CCK, PYY and GLP-1. We learned about these in the Appetite Satisfaction section of the Introduction; recall that these chemical messengers signal the hypothalamus to suppress your appetite, leaving you feeling satisfied. Dietary fat also slows the rate at which food empties from the stomach. Meals containing sufficient dietary fat help delay gastric emptying, helping you feel full longer.

In addition to the three hormones mentioned above, newer research reveals fascinating evidence linking dietary fat to appetite suppression through a signaling molecule known as oleoylethanolamide (OEA). Produced by the small intestine, OEA works in an interesting way to help limit food intake. This signal works on a long-term scale, prolonging the length of time before hunger returns. By staying fuller for longer, chances are you'll take in fewer calories through a decrease in your meal frequency. Eating enough fat is the only way to produce enough OEA to keep hunger at bay for hour after hour; carbohydrate and protein intake don't contribute to OEA production.

Most gut hormones reduce meal size, giving you the signal "we're good, put down the fork," but OEA lengthens the amount of time between meals, so you can be off living your life for several hours before hunger comes back. Anyone who has followed a low-fat meal plan before knows that truly forgetting about eating is not a common experience when you're cutting fat grams to a minimum.

Geek Tip: OEA also alters fuel metabolism through activation of the PPARalpha transcription factor. This transcription factor modifies gene expression, priming the entire body to switch more toward burning fat than carbohydrate. Bottom line: if you eat more fat, your body adjusts to burn more fat.

So by eating enough fat, you can get more satisfied at meals, go longer between meals without being hungry and activate genes which turn up your body's ability to mobilize stored fat and torch it.

Eating enough dietary fat also effectively protects against hypoglycemia—commonly experienced as raging hunger due to falling blood glucose. The amount of available fuel sources in your bloodstream impact the return of hunger several hours after you eat. Low-fat meals may leave you feeling just fine in the short term, but three to four hours after the meal you might experience excessive hunger and potential symptoms such as shakiness, lightheadedness and feeling chilly. Having a moderate amount of fat with a meal results in greater circulating energy available for hours after eating and better appetite control for the same amount of calories. Plus, your co-workers will thank you for never getting "hangry" again!

Time to update your tracker. You've got all the info you need; now it's time for practice.

HABIT	1	2	3	4	5	6	7	8	9	10	11	12	13	14
Eat 3 or 4 meals without snacking														
Hunger Mastery (hunger for 30–60 minutes before eating)														
Eat just enough at each meal														
Eat mostly (or all) whole foods														
Eat at least 6 cups of vegetables														
Reduce or eliminate liquid calories														
30–40 grams of protein at each meal														
15 grams of fat approx. at each meal														

LEAN HABIT 9:
MEET YOUR CARBOHYDRATE NEEDS WISELY

WHAT TO DO

I recommend a moderate amount of carbohydrates, and that you get most of them from non-starchy vegetables and fruit. These low-glycemic sources are lower in calorie density than grains, beans or sugars and are higher in nutrient density. Getting most of your carbohydrates from non-starchy vegetables and fruit, with a smaller contribution from non-starchy whole grains and beans, will help you enjoy a high level of appetite satisfaction and nutrition per calorie, without any food being off-limits.

INDIVIDUALIZING CARBOHYDRATE INTAKE

After years of working with hundreds of clients, I can tell you that there is some trial and error involved in finding the perfect carbohydrate level for optimal happiness, physical well-being and fat loss for any given client. Individual tailoring is always part of the process, and working with clients one-on-one allows me to take personal preference into account when deciding where to suggest adding or subtracting foods. A moderate carbohydrate intake can be achieved equally well with small, frequent portions of starchy foods as with infrequent, larger portions. Additionally, some people prefer the high-volume satisfaction of eating only fruit and vegetables for carbohydrates and choose grains and potatoes rarely, if at all.

My client Erin, for example, really enjoyed her morning oatmeal with blueberries, plus some cooked grain or potato at dinner with her family, so we made sure to keep those in place while paring out extra calories and carbohydrates elsewhere in her day and working on portion sizes. Erin made great progress with fat loss eating these every single day, and felt a ton of relief that she didn't have to part with these foods just because they were high in carbohydrates. Her previous attempts at fat loss had always been a struggle because she felt like she *shouldn't* have starchy carbohydrates twice in one day. Other clients of mine consume one or two portions of starch each day but include more on hard workout days. Some clients consume a side portion of starch with every meal. And they make progress just as rapidly. So there's more than one way to do it, and you can always consult with a One By One Nutrition coach if you want help in personalizing your carbohydrate intake.

WHY IT'S WORTH IT

Since you've already been practicing loading up on lots of fruits and vegetables, you're already taking in some carbohydrates, likely close to 100 grams a day from those alone. Is this enough or do you need to add more? The answer is … it depends. Mostly, your carbohydrate needs are determined by how physically active you are.

Of the three major macronutrients, carbohydrates are the least appetite satisfying in the acute sense. But, there are plenty of reasons to include extra carbohydrates above and beyond fruits and vegetables by eating more carbohydrate-dense foods like whole grains, sweet potatoes, winter squash and beans. Extra carbohydrates improve athletic performance and recovery, aid in muscle growth and help prevent overtraining syndrome. Some of your favorite foods may be carbohydrate-dense, and enjoyment is also an important thing to take into account! Remember, suffering is optional; I'd prefer you enjoy your meals as much as possible.

You read in an earlier lesson how low-fat and high-fat diets are undesirable for attaining health and a lean body composition; well, carbohydrates are a similar story, in that neither extreme of low or high intake is ideal. At intake levels that are too low, you're likely to be plagued by cravings, have diminished energy and athletic capacity and weaken your immune system. But too many carbohydrates can prevent weight-loss success, so it's worth finding the best amount for you.

"WHERE DO STARCHY FOODS FIT IN?"

The short answer is: it depends on your appetite, results and how much exercise you do.

The current habits you're practicing have already put a lot on your plate, literally. At each meal, you should be taking in two to three cups of vegetables, with some fruit here and there. (Substantial weight and volume of food: Check!) You're aiming for 30 to 40 grams of protein, and you know you need a minimum of 15 grams of appetite-satisfying fat. (Protein and fat-triggered satiety hormones accounted for: Check!) You might be satisfied on all that already. So in the name of mastering Eat Just Enough, you're done.

But if you've *still* got room before you hit your stopping point of Eating Just Enough, you'll want to eat a bit more. Given that you've covered your nutritional bases for appetite satisfaction, **any** whole food will do. You could simply eat a few more bites of meat or vegetables or fruit, but it's fine to include something starchy like rice, bread or quinoa. Just bear in mind:

- Lower-GI (glyemic index) foods (sweet potatoes, oatmeal, quinoa, winter squash, fruit and beans) are better choices than high-glycemic foods (most cold cereals, bagels, crackers, candy, granola bars and desserts), so choose them most of the time.

- To lose weight, you want to stop eating at Just Enough, so after eating vegetables, protein and fat, you probably don't need more than a small side portion of grain, beans or potato.

- If you exercise a lot, you are likely to be able to lose weight with more starchy foods in your diet, even including them with every meal. If you exercise less, however, you need fewer carbohydrates and calories, so try adding fruits or vegetables instead of starches at least some of the time if you need a bit more food to get satisfied. More on that in the next habit.

The important message here is *not* to tell yourself "don't eat white rice, but brown rice is fine" or "white potatoes are high glycemic and therefore not allowed," and I certainly don't want you to scour the Internet for lists of high- and low-glycemic-load foods and start swearing off anything that is higher than a certain number. Drawing a line in the sand or demonizing food types is a cognitive shortcut for easy decision-making, but it can rob you of seeing the whole picture.

Better than rules, I want to impart understanding with these lessons. I hope you understand that certain carbohydrate-containing foods have health and weight-loss benefits (whole grains over refined grains, for example), so it's advantageous if your overall pattern of consumption favors those foods. But there's not a dire problem with having a serving of white rice or white potato occasionally in a whole-food-based diet with overall moderate carbohydrates and fat. Your favorite foods can fit. The nutritional difference between ⅓ cup of brown rice and ⅓ cup of white rice is really negligible in the context of a whole day, so don't let specifying food types distract you from the overall important factor for weight loss: quantity. Many people inadvertently stall their progress by becoming overly focused on avoiding white flour and sugar while eating more calories than they need in quinoa and sweet potatoes.

HOW IT WORKS

Not enough carbohydrate impacts physical performance and well-being. You may experience some negative effects if you cut your carbohydrate intake too low. Primarily, training tolerance and recovery after exercise suffer if the diet provides inadequate carbohydrate. You might notice that after workouts you want to go lie down and not do anything for a long while, or that you feel spent before you even complete your workout (like you're running out of gas early). While weight training you'll notice three things:

• You won't be able to do as many sets.

• You will need extra rest between your sets.

- As you do your sets you won't get as many reps in the later sets as usual. For example if you did squats and normally performed eight, seven, six, six, five reps per set; you might only get eight, six, four, three in the carb-depleted state.

Additional signs of inadequate carbohydrate intake include having a harder time falling asleep and/or staying asleep. You may notice you get more frequent colds or infections than most people. Too-low carbohydrate intake can lead to increased carbohydrate cravings (sweet or starchy foods) and decreased quality of life.

How low is "too low" for you can vary substantially based on your activity level, genetics and the type of exercise you do. For most people who are moderately active (exercising three to five times per week), these symptoms commonly appear as total carbohydrate intake drops below 100 grams per day. But in people who are highly active, signs of inadequate carbohydrate intake can be seen at 200 grams a day. In the Olympic athletes I work with, four to five hours of training per day results in carbohydrate needs of over 300 grams per day. Rather than counting up numbers, just as you've learned to do with your appetite, the best way to get the right amount of carbohydrates is to tune in to your body. If you notice the signs and symptoms mentioned above, try adding more carbohydrate to your meals to see if it alleviates your problems.

EXCESS CARBOHYDRATE FAVORS WEIGHT GAIN AND METABOLIC DISEASE

Carbohydrates provide less satisfaction per calorie than protein or fat, so if we remember our overall mission is to get into a calorie deficit as comfortably as possible, we want enough carbohydrates to prevent the problems described above, but not much more. Any extra carbohydrates above that are just extra calories that don't provide much satiety.

The increase in carbohydrate content of the North American diet was paralleled by an increase in calorie consumption and obesity rates. This is not surprising, given that some research indicates that the higher the carbohydrate content of someone's diet, the more calories they are likely to eat and the more they are likely to weigh. In clinical trials, reducing the amount of total dietary carbohydrate has been shown to be more effective for weight loss than reducing dietary fat, particularly for insulin-resistant people.

CARBOHYDRATE TYPES MATTER TOO

Certain types of carbohydrate have been consistently associated with obesity and health. Intake of sugar-sweetened beverages, refined grain products, potatoes and refined bread have been associated with excess weight and/or greater waist circumference. Dietary fiber has been associated in many studies with lower BMI, smaller waist circumference, lower body fat and weight reduction over time.

High-GI (glycemic index) foods break down rapidly and cause greater elevations in blood glucose after a meal. Low-GI foods break down slowly, causing a milder rise in blood glucose that declines gradually over several hours. Choosing a low glycemic diet pattern means choosing low-GI foods, keeping total carbohydrates moderate and is generally better for health and weight loss. Glycemic load is a term that takes into account the glycemic index of a food as well as the total amount of carbohydrate. Thus, a tiny amount of a high-GI food still has a low glycemic load.

Calorie for calorie, eating a high-glycemic-index food causes more insulin to be released than eating a low-glycemic-index food. But the dramatic rise in blood insulin leads to rapid clearing of the glucose from the bloodstream, leaving blood sugar lower three to four hours after a high-GI meal than after a low-GI meal. While many factors contribute to hunger, research supports that low blood sugar is a powerful initiator of hunger. When your blood sugar falls, you're going to feel compelled to seek food and eat it now. (This effect is seen whether blood glucose reaches a low absolute value or simply sustains a decline, even if it never dips below the normal range.) This is consistent with studies showing that high-glycemic-index meals lead to overeating later, whereas low-glycemic meals have been repeatedly shown to produce greater satisfaction, delayed hunger return and less food intake at subsequent meals. In fact, even after controlling for total calorie intake, higher-glycemic diets have been associated with greater body mass index (BMI). This may be due to the appetite-stimulating and fat-storage-promoting effects of higher insulin levels.

MRI STUDIES OF THE HUMAN BRAIN SHOW THAT A SINGLE HIGH-GLYCEMIC MEAL SELECTIVELY STIMULATES BRAIN REGIONS ASSOCIATED WITH REWARD AND CRAVING FOR SEVERAL HOURS AFTER THE MEAL.

People eating low-glycemic diets experience less metabolic adaptation during weight loss than those eating high-glycemic diets, with preservation of resting metabolic rate and circulating levels of the hormone leptin. Decline in leptin level is one of the challenges that makes it harder to keep losing weight as a person get leaner; the more leptin levels fall, the less you feel like moving. Thyroid hormone output falls when leptin is diminished, and appetite is increased. So if choosing low-glycemic meals can prevent that all from happening and preserve your leptin level during weight loss, it sounds worth it to me!

Aside from being beneficial from a fat-loss perspective, it's worth mentioning that paying attention to the quantity and quality of carbohydrates you eat is a health matter too. Higher-carbohydrate diets, and especially high-glycemic-index and high-glycemic-load diets, have been associated with increased risk of hemorrhagic and ischemic stroke. Glycemic load has been associated with increased risk for certain cancers, including breast, prostate, colorectal, rectal and pancreatic, as well as the risk of developing type 2 diabetes. Eating more rapidly digestible carbohydrates has also been linked to elevations in C-reactive protein, a marker of inflammation and risk factor for heart disease.

Interestingly, functional MRI studies of the human brain show that a single high-glycemic meal selectively stimulates brain regions associated with reward and craving for several hours after the meal. This craving stimulation effect is significantly lower after a lower-GI meal equal in calories and macronutrients. So if you feel like once you start eating sweets and baked goods you only crave them more, you're exactly right. Switching from sugary processed sweets like candy to slower-digesting, more balanced treats that don't spike blood glucose as dramatically can help you break any "addictive" powers that sugar has over you.

YOU'VE GOT A HEAD START

I've reviewed research in this lesson that shows limiting glycemic load to be favorable for health and fat loss. And I'd like to point out that the habits you already have in place from prior lessons have already helped you take strides toward a low-glycemic diet. Eating mostly or all whole foods means that many high-glycemic foods such as rice cakes, muffins and cake are already minimized in your diet. As for foods that are unprocessed yet still have a high-glycemic index, such as white potatoes for example, the overall glycemic load is moderated by portion control. If you are practicing eating enough protein, fat and vegetables, there isn't room for oversized servings of starches if you are stopping after Eating Just Enough.

Update your habit tracker with the following habit: "Choose low-glycemic starches in small portions if extra carbohydrates are needed."

HABIT	1	2	3	4	5	6	7	8	9	10	11	12	13	14
Eat 3 or 4 meals without snacking														
Hunger Mastery (hunger for 30–60 minutes before eating)														
Eat just enough at each meal														
Eat mostly (or all) whole foods														
Eat at least 6 cups of vegetables														
Reduce or eliminate liquid calories														
30–40 grams of protein at each meal														
15 grams of fat approx. at each meal														
Choose low-glycemic starches in small portions if extra carbohydrates are needed														

LEAN HABIT 10:
ADAPT YOUR CARBOHYDRATE STRATEGY FOR YOUR EXERCISE GOALS

As you read in the prior lesson, carbohydrates are not nearly as powerful as protein and fat at eliciting short-term satiety signals from the gut, but that doesn't make them "bad" by any means! **Carbohydrates have other important functions, one of those being the preferred fuel for intense exercise.** In this section, I'll mention some special adjustments to your carbohydrate intake which are beneficial if you are an athlete with a competitive season. If you're exercising mainly for fat loss, a little carbohydrate strategy around your workouts can help you get closer to your goals too.

WHAT TO DO

For competitive athletes, I recommend that during the competitive season and when training volume is highest, glycogen replenishment should be prioritized by consuming carbohydrates before, during and after exercise as needed to maintain peak performance. That means fat loss takes a back seat to fueling performance.

For noncompetitive exercisers looking to reduce fat, I recommend consuming a mixed meal after intense exercise, with protein, vegetables and fat as previously described for appetite management, plus a serving of starchy carbohydrates. Don't get too hung up on grams or serving sizes of the carbohydrates, just aim for about a handful of cooked whole grains, cereal, winter squash, potato or sweet potato. You can increase or decrease the amount depending on your fat loss progress and exercise intensity and duration on a given day. For the most rapid success with fat loss, aim for the lowest amount of additional carbohydrates that leaves you without the problems described in the previous lesson.

THE BEST WAY TO KNOW IS TO EVALUATE YOUR OWN EXPERIENCE. IF YOU ARE FEELING GREAT AND YOUR RESULTS ARE COMING ALONG, DON'T FIX ANYTHING BECAUSE NOTHING IS BROKEN.

If some or all of your exercise sessions are low intensity, such as walking or yoga, you may find that you don't need to include more carbohydrates in your post-workout meal than those you obtain from fruits and vegetables (which you're already including each time you eat, right?). The best way to know is to evaluate your own experience. If you are feeling great and your results are coming along, don't fix anything because nothing is broken. However, if you are feeling fatigued for hours after your training, or having strong cravings for sweet or starchy foods in the hours after your workouts that lead to slipups and eating additional calories later in the day, try adding additional carbohydrates to your post-exercise meal to see if this alleviates the trouble.

IF PERFORMANCE AND RECOVERY ARE YOUR GOAL

If you are a competitive athlete, at certain times in the year you may need to prioritize your athletic performance over maximizing fat loss. What you eat before a Tuesday night spin class doesn't matter so much, but if you're trying to run your best half marathon or help your soccer team win a championship, you can get a boost from extra complex carbohydrates above and beyond the moderate amount I've recommended for fat loss in the previous habit. Consuming carbohydrates before, during and after exercise has been shown to help augment performance and hasten replenishment of depleted glycogen stores.

Before: Consuming one to three grams of carbohydrate per kilogram of bodyweight in the one to four hours before competition is recommended to maximize athletic performance, especially for endurance athletes such as runners, cyclists and triathletes.

During: In events lasting longer than 90 minutes, replenishing carbohydrates at the rate of 30 to 60 grams per hour helps you keep going at your strongest.

After: Eating carbohydrates (preferably along with a smaller amount of protein) helps your body rebuild depleted glycogen stores, recover from the workout or race and avoid post-exercise immune suppression.

IS IT REALLY CRITICAL TO EAT RIGHT AWAY AFTER EXERCISE?

The importance of getting **immediate** post-exercise nutrition has been somewhat overstated by well-intentioned personal trainers, leaving some fitness enthusiasts convinced that the urgency of drinking a recovery shake warrants sprinting to the locker room to hastily chug a chalky drink, lest their whole workout be utterly wasted if they miss the critical 20-minute window.

Getting immediate post-workout nutrition is most important for athletes who train twice in a day, and for athletes who train after an overnight fast who are in a particularly catabolic state, but these aren't common circumstances. Most people are not training twice a day, and have eaten in the several hours before their workout. For athletes training once per day, there is evidence that as long as 24-hour carbohydrate intake is sufficient, carbohydrates don't necessarily have to be forced into any arbitrary "post-workout" window. So for most of us, no need to panic if it takes 30 minutes to get home and prep something to eat.

IF FAT LOSS IS YOUR GOAL

Most of my clients are not competitive, and they don't have to worry about qualifying for the Olympics. They are everyday gym-goers who want to lose as much fat as possible. For fat loss, it's not such a big deal if glycogen replenishment isn't absolutely maximized, you just need to get into a calorie deficit most days and stay happy. You might think then that it doesn't matter if you recover from workouts, or that you're best off skipping eating after a workout so you don't undo the calorie deficit you created by sweating through time on the treadmill. But you'd be wrong; skipping carbohydrates in your post-workout meal (or skipping your post-workout meal altogether) is not a good idea, even if your only goal is losing fat.

One of the reasons I encourage my fat loss clients to eat a meal containing extra carbohydrates after exercise is to prevent an uncontrollable appetite later. Exercising hard and not fully refueling afterward makes a person hungry. Really hungry. In addition to hunger pangs, not eating much after a strenuous workout commonly leaves a person vulnerable to feeling mental strain, including twinges of deprivation and entitlement later in the day. In my years of working with clients in private practice, I've observed that investing calories into a satisfying and nutritious post-workout meal does great things for clients' fat-loss results, even if indirectly, by preventing strong cravings and spontaneous justifications from luring you into overeating later. Adding a serving of starchy food like bread, oats or quinoa to a post-workout meal may contribute an extra 100 to 200 calories, but prevent you from falling into "I earned this" thinking that leads to eating 500 calories of popcorn that evening. In my experience, shortchanging your body on carbohydrates after a hard workout often results in a strong appetite increase and powerful carbohydrate cravings in the three to six hours following your exercise.

Research shows that this isn't just my observation, it has been demonstrated in controlled studies. Both aerobic training and weightlifting use up stored carbohydrates, and replenishing those carbohydrates during or soon after training results in better hunger control and less calorie intake over the course of the whole day.

If you exercise hard regularly, update your habit tracker with this new habit: "Follow intense exercise with a meal containing starchy carbohydrate." Note: if you don't exercise intensely on a given day, feel free to record "n/a" for that day.

HABIT	1	2	3	4	5	6	7	8	9	10	11	12	13	14
Eat 3 or 4 meals without snacking														
Hunger Mastery (hunger for 30–60 minutes before eating)														
Eat just enough at each meal														
Eat mostly (or all) whole foods														
Eat at least 6 cups of vegetables														
Reduce or eliminate liquid calories														
30–40 grams of protein at each meal														
15 grams of fat approx. at each meal														
Choose low-glycemic starches in small portions if extra carbohydrates are needed														
Follow intense exercise with a meal containing starchy carbohydrate, if applicable														

LEAN HABIT 11:

BE 100 PERCENT AWARE OF THE TREATS YOU EAT

WHAT TO DO

It all starts with awareness. **The first step is to keep track of how many treats you eat in a typical stretch of two weeks.** No judgment is involved—simply observe. You don't need to log calories or grams of sugar or anything like that; a simple tally will do.

Before I go further about their place in a fat-loss diet, let's define what I mean by "treats." I use this term to include high-calorie but low-nutrient foods (such as desserts, added sugars, refined bread products, potato chips, candy, muffins, ice cream), as well as alcoholic beverages and fried foods. Basically, treats are things we consume chiefly for pleasure and taste that have higher calories for their satiety value and nutrition than other things we might eat.

It's an important skill to be fully aware of every single thing you eat, and if you get a little squirmy at the idea of writing down every bite and nibble you take, be aware that you probably will benefit more from this exercise than other people. If you do feel some resistance, it might be because you're afraid to see how many treats you eat, or you want to make a case for yourself that the small bits and pieces you eat don't count so you shouldn't have to write them down. You might even feel a little angry. This resistance comes from judgment—if you remember that having treats is fine, and the goal is just to observe, it will be easier to let go of the judgment, and the resistance. It doesn't matter if you have five or 500 treats in the next two weeks, what matters is that you own them. Don't hide them from consciousness by coming up with an excuse to not log it.

This information is only for you. And it's a big step to first be honest with yourself. Don't be afraid to let yourself see in black and white how much of this stuff you eat. It doesn't make you a bad person, it's just food.

Many people are surprised to some degree when they first do a two-week observation period to see how many treats they actually consume. It can be eye-opening and sobering to realize that you actually take in 10, 20 or 30 treats in a two-week span when it feels like you only have them "occasionally." However, once the wincing stops, it's also frequently reassuring for clients to see that they take in so many extra calories currently, because it leaves a margin to comfortably reduce them (and see more weight loss) without hitting zero! I point out to clients whose weight loss has stalled that it's a beautiful thing actually to see that you are taking in a lot of calories from sugars or other "extras" because it means you will have plenty of them left in your diet after choosing just a few less.

WHY IT'S WORTH IT

Most of us want to eat something less than nutritious every now and then. But a frequent intake of high-calorie, low-nutrient foods contributes to body fat storage and poor health. Swearing off your favorite treats or declaring certain foods off-limits until you reach a weight-loss goal can produce feelings of restriction and denial, and often leads to unfavorable outcomes. Mastering this habit is the first step toward discovering a sustainable balance that will work long term to manage treats, so that you make progress toward your goals without feeling deprived.

HOW IT WORKS

If weight loss was all that mattered in the world, I'd say "stop eating treats" and this would be a very short lesson. But fat loss is not all there is to life, and complete abstinence from these foods isn't necessary to be lean and healthy! In fact, accepting deprivation works against you, because if you're sacrificing a lot and expending lots of effort to stick to your eating plan, you can't keep it up for long, certainly not the rest of your life. (If you've tried to give up all your favorite foods, you might be nodding your head right now.) I prefer pleasant and sustainable weight loss, so it's my goal to figure out how many treats can fit into my clients' diets while allowing for weight loss. And then I expect them to enjoy them happily and guilt free!

Whatever system you are using to keep track of your habit practice, now's the time to add your eleventh habit: "Keep track of treats." Below that, add rows for tracking the following different categories of treats.

HABIT	1	2	3	4	5	6	7	8	9	10	11	12	13	14
Keep track of treats														
Alchohol or caloric drinks (1 per drink)														
Sweets, desserts, candy (1 per cupcake, slice of cake, cookie, ounce of chocolate, ½ cup ice cream or frozen yogurt)														
Deep-fried food: chips, tortilla chips (1 per handful)														
Sugar added to coffee, tea, cereal or yogurt (1 per tsp)														
Processed foods (cereal bars, protein bars, ramen, etc.)														

You'll notice that even if you have really small quantities, such as one packet of sugar, I want you to record them. A single packet of sugar is itself absolutely not going to mean much for weight loss, but a bit of this and a bit of that does add up and can play a significant role in your progress, so be sure to capture everything. If you have less than a serving, half a handful of chips for example, write "0.5" rather than ignoring it. Fight the urge to disown or discount any of your food choices. They all count. And I'll say it again, there's nothing wrong with enjoying treats! If you have a mint after dinner, write it down. Mine a chunk of brownie out of the ice cream carton in the freezer? Write it down. The biggest thing you are gaining now is awareness.

Some clients question viewing protein bars as treats because they seem like healthier choices than candy and because they have some nutrients added to them. I advise keeping track of them not because they are necessarily a problem, but because they *can* be an obstacle to weight loss. As a reminder: writing something down doesn't mean it's "bad" or has to go, it's just information.

Many protein bars are dense sources of calories and aren't as filling as protein from whole foods. I advise my clients that protein and nutrition bars fall into two categories, and to take necessary precautions with each type. There are protein bars that are dangerous because they taste good, and ones are dangerous because they don't taste that good. Protein bars that taste great potentially introduce extra calories because, like other sweet foods, we're likely to eat them for the taste, even if we aren't truly hungry. When I used to pack a peanut butter–chocolate protein bar with my lunch each day, you bet I ate that sucker after my salad every day because it was sweet, crispy and tasty—if my salad filled me up, I'm sure I would have eaten it anyway.

Bars that don't taste that good cause trouble too. After we've eaten one, we may feel deprived of a more filling meal (and reach for more food), or we may want something else to get the nasty aftertaste out of our mouths. We might feel spiteful that we spent $3.49 on a chemical-tasting brick when the Snickers right next to it was only $0.89. We might also feel virtuous for choosing such a "healthy" snack, even though it was 300 calories, and justify having an extra slice of pizza or fries with dinner. I've also observed that clients who eat protein bars as desserts in place of "real sweets" often end up taking in just as many calories but feel like they're sacrificing taste; sometimes they even end up bingeing on the real thing on the weekend after depriving themselves all week. In that case, reducing calories can be achieved by losing the calorie-dense bars and eating small portions of the genuine thing. In any event, it won't hurt you to gain awareness of all the types of treats you eat, including protein bars.

Once you've recorded your treats tally for two weeks, you've got some numbers to look at.

HABIT	1	2	3	4	5	6	7	8	9	10	11	12	13	14
Eat 3 or 4 meals without snacking														
Hunger Mastery (hunger for 30–60 min before eating)														
Eat just enough at each meal														
Eat mostly (or all) whole foods														
Eat at least 6 cups of vegetables														
Reduce or eliminate liquid calories														
30–40 grams of protein at each meal														
15 grams of fat approx. at each meal														
Choose low glycemic starches in small portions if extra carbohydrates are needed														
Follow intense exercise with a meal containing starchy carbohydrate, if applicable														
Keep track of treats														
Alchohol or caloric drinks (1 per drink)														
Sweets, desserts, candy (1 per cupcake, slice of cake, cookie, ounce of chocolate, ½ cup ice cream or frozen yogurt)														
Deep-fried food: chips, tortilla chips (1 per handful)														
Sugar added to coffee, tea, cereal or yogurt (1 per tsp)														
Processed foods (cereal bars, protein bars, ramen, etc.)														

LEAN HABIT 12:
MANAGE TREATS WITH AN EYE ON YOUR GOALS

If you add those numbers up, you'll get a total of, let's say, 34 treats. If during the two weeks you recorded those 34 treats you lost weight (0.5 to 1 pound per week), we might just decide that staying at the same level is a good goal, since it's working. That was easy. If it ain't broke, don't fix it. Keep doing whatever you're doing. How simple is that?

If your weight loss is slower than 0.5 to 1 pound per week, and you'd like to accelerate it, trimming back on the treats is a very effective place to start. Here's the important part—dial them back, don't cut them out.

Here are some strategies to help you reduce excess calories from treats, lose weight *and* keep the smile on your face and your "deprivation meter" close to zero.

WHAT TO DO

If you want to see greater weight loss than you currently are achieving, decide how much of a reduction in your treats is realistic without being overly severe. Consider these four tips in this lesson when deciding on a number of treats to aim for in the next two weeks.

1. Consider what makes a treat "worth it" or "not worth it." The whole purpose of eating treats is pleasure, so they should be pleasurable enough to be worth taking a small step back from weight loss. If you think about the many types of treat, you'll probably agree that they run on a spectrum: some are amazing and some are definitely not amazing. You might not like store-bought cookies or apple pie for example, but swoon over imported dark chocolate or a glass of fine Italian wine. If you think back to all the treats tallied on your tracker, one or two of them might not have been highly enjoyable, but more accurately described as "so-so" or "just okay." Paring out the so-so or just okay treats can save you considerable calories, often enough to lose weight. If you can't tell at first glance whether a treat is really delicious or not, let the first bite be your test. If it's not amazing, don't eat any more. This treat strategy can contribute to your lifetime leanness while still keeping lots of enjoyable experiences in your life.

Besides the food itself, other circumstances contribute to how enjoyable a treat experience is. A hot August afternoon trip to the ice cream parlor with your kids is very different from scarfing ice cream from the carton, standing in front of the freezer at 3 a.m. because you're angry the neighbor's barking dog woke you up. The setting, your mood, the amount of time you have to enjoy it and even your intention when eating it can all make the difference. Think for a moment of what makes a treat "worth it" to you, as well as what would make one "not worth it." Your list might look like this:

Worth it: dark chocolate, homemade cookies, fine wine, when I'm calm and have time to savor it slowly, when I can share it with someone, when it's about having something tasty and not an emotional reason.

Not worth it: cheap or milk chocolate, anything with raisins, anything in the office break room, eating it when I'm in a rush, when I'm driving, when I'm sad and seeking comfort or procrastinating. If I'm eating it "just because it's there."

Deciding to only eat treats that are on your personal "worth it list" is a way to raise the bar. Keep the best ones, don't settle and you'll likely find the total number of treats manageable to reduce by at least a little.

2. Eat mindfully and savor each and every bite with your full attention. To repeat, the whole purpose of having treats is pleasure, so if you are absentmindedly eating while doing something else or your mind wanders elsewhere, you won't get the full enjoyment and may seek a larger quantity to make up for the diluted experience. Ideally, we wouldn't rush when eating anything, but it's *especially* critical when you're choosing something just for its taste, so slow down and enjoy it. Smell it, notice its color and texture, pay attention to how it feels in your mouth. Committing to always eating treats mindfully can further help you get greater enjoyment from each bite, preventing deprivation while you pare back the total amount of treats.

3. Think of portion size and frequency as separate variables to modify. The impact of any food on your overall diet can be expressed as portion size times frequency. That means reducing either portion or frequency is an effective way of reducing the impact of a particular food, as long as the other one stays the same. Some people find it's easier to switch to smaller portions, and some find it's easier to just have treats less often but keep the portion the same. In my experience people are pretty evenly split, so feel free to do whichever seems more manageable to you.

Here's an example: if you normally consume four drinks a night every Saturday and Sunday, but want to trim your alcohol intake, consider if you would prefer to modify the portion size or the frequency. To modify portion size, you could commit to stopping at two or three drinks per night. If you opted instead to alter the frequency, you could decide to drink only one night per week (without increasing the amount) or only every other weekend.

Similarly, if you see that your treats tracker reflects eating three cookies a night, you could try to reduce to two mindfully eaten cookies, or just not have cookies every other night and have tea instead.

4. Increase other sources of fun and relaxation. Sometimes eating treats is part of a wind-down routine after work, a fun escape on weekends or some "me time" at the end of a long day. Reducing the number of treats you consume doesn't mean cutting back on fun or denying yourself much-needed relaxation! If anything, try to find *more* joy and rest in non-food ways. Choose other activities to relax, like taking quiet time with a book, a walk outside or a conversation with your spouse. If you think none of those would fit in your schedule, remind yourself that if you would have taken time to eat, you can take a few minutes to care for yourself instead.

Write your goal for total treat intake over the next two weeks in your tracker and continue recording your intake of these foods to stay aware. If most of your treats are coming from a certain category, you may choose to simply work on bringing that category down and keeping the others the same, such as "Goal: less than 15 servings of sweets." Or you can set an overall goal, such as "Fewer than 25 treats total." Here's an example of our sample tracker, reflecting that the user set a goal to bring her total treats down to 25:

Hunger Mastery (hunger for 30–60 minutes before eating)												
Eat just enough at each meal												
Eat mostly (or all) whole foods												
Eat at least 6 cups of vegetables												
Reduce or eliminate liquid calories												
30–40 grams of protein at each meal												
15 grams of fat approx. at each meal												
Choose low-glycemic starches in small portions if extra carbohydrates are needed												
Follow intense exercise with a meal containing starchy carbohydrate, if applicable												
Keep track of treats (Goal for these 2 weeks: <25 total)												
Alchohol or caloric drinks (1 per drink)												
Sweets, desserts, candy (1 per cupcake, slice of cake, cookie, ounce of chocolate, ½ cup ice cream or frozen yogurt)												
Deep-fried food: chips, tortilla chips (1 per handful)												
Sugar added to coffee, tea, cereal or yogurt (1 per tsp)												
Processed foods (cereal bars, protein bars, ramen, etc.)												

You are likely to adjust and refine your treats tally over time. If you notice your weight-loss progress has stalled, it is one of the first places to troubleshoot. Once you've reached your goal weight, it also serves as an important yardstick for showing you what level of fun, indulgent eating you need to maintain your weight loss and not regain.

SUCCESS-BOOSTING TIP: AVOID EXCESSIVE DEBATE

Getting embroiled in lengthy emotional disagreements is never pleasant, but it's especially pesky when it's *you* on both sides! Here's what I mean: you show up at your friend's Super Bowl party and set your sensible tray of veggies and hummus among the extensive spread of food. You spot some shrimp cocktail, and you're thinking "Sweet! I can get some lean protein there, nosh on a pile of veggies and hummus, take a handful of whole grain crackers and I'm set! I don't care for those greasy wings anyway." But then you spot the tray of brownies. Thick, fudgy, walnut-studded blocks of temptation, and your palms start to sweat. Your mind starts going, "I want one. I can't have one. Yes, I can. But I shouldn't, not if I want to lose weight. Well, one won't hurt. Yes it will. Just walk away. Eat some celery…"

An hour and a half later, you have eaten the veggies and hummus and shrimp you intended to, but your mind is still fixated on the brownies, despite consuming an entire two-liter bottle of diet soda to try to make your sweet tooth shut up. While the other guests are cheering on the teams, your mind is keeping stats on precisely who has eaten a brownie, who has had two and you officially hate your friend's thin husband who has had *four*. Your internal debate is clashing harder than the gridiron helmets on the screen. "I've held out this long, but I'll never make it through the second half. I'm eating one. No! Don't do it! You'll regret it!" You keep looking at the tray, thinking that if you pick the smallest brownie, it won't be so bad, or if you just break off a piece…you see other people looking happy and enjoying the game while you stew. You are tired of being unhappy, tired of not getting what you want. Resentment builds. You head over to the table, already feeling like a failure for giving in before you get there, so you shut out the shameful feelings and go into numb autopilot, grabbing one brownie with each hand and quickly darting into the kitchen so nobody sees you scarfing them down.

If this experience sounds familiar, you know that it often doesn't end with two brownies, and the chances of you enjoying the remainder the party are slim to none. More likely, you don't feel satisfied after the first round, and want to eat and eat and eat, as you feel increasingly horrible about yourself and your behavior. What happened? Why does a seemingly normal social situation end in a dozen brownies and a silent car ride home during which your baffled husband tries to figure out what on earth has gotten you so upset that you look like you're about to cry? *Maybe she just really, really doesn't like football?*

The problem is not that you have a character flaw or weakness. The problem is not that you "can't control yourself" or that you are "addicted to sugar." The problem is the food debate.

Georgie's Law: the duration and emotional amplitude of your internal debate over eating a treat is proportional to the urgency and desire for massive quantities you'll feel.

In other words, the more minutes you spend vacillating back and forth over eating (or not eating) a food item, and the more impassioned you get over it, the more likely you are to consume a metric ton of it. As a food debate progresses, the craving and tension you feel become less and less about the actual food and more about relieving the stress of the deliberation. More than eating a baked good, you just want to escape the indecision over eating the baked good! And if you decide even for one second "I'm going to eat it," it's like a doorway to feeling better just opened. So you sprint for it, consuming the contentious food hastily and in half awareness, as you fight to get it in before the stinging guilt sets in. The food is hardly ever satisfying because after all, you inhaled it and were primarily acting to escape the debate, not enjoy a sensory thrill. Since you're left unsatisfied, it's enticing to just keep going, thinking that it simply will take more of the food to feel better.

As you can see, your thoughts are what drive compulsion or craving. It's not a random thing like a hailstorm that just happens to you (and never happens to some others).

You can learn to opt out of this thought pattern and stop suffering massive compulsions to eat all the ice cream. Once you stop giving yourself hailstorms in the form of emotional food debates, losing weight is easier.

The experience can be "I ate it, I enjoyed it, I moved on." Or, you can choose to pass on it, put it out of your mind and go back to the rest of your life. The key isn't whether you say yes or no, but to make a decision and be done with it. Recognize that no one food decision is all that important, and there is no right or wrong way to use your treat budget. If you get twitchy and can feel tension rising about whether to eat something or not, remember what will really make you feel better is not the food, but ending the debate so your mind can be at peace.

LEAN HABIT 13:
SHAPE YOUR SOCIAL AND PHYSICAL ENVIRONMENT

WHY IT'S WORTH IT

The physical items surrounding you have a powerful influence on you, including your food choices. **Modifying your food environment is a key skill in making a permanent lifestyle change and drastically reduces the amount of effort and willpower you'll need to exert.** I want leanness for you to be as effortless as possible. In addition to the physical environment you live and work in, the social context of your life is very influential on your food decisions. Changing your eating habits to help you reach your goals is more pleasant and permanent when you have support (or at least, minimal objections) from your family and friends.

HOW IT WORKS

Physical Environment

The influence of any particular food on your decision-making is impacted by its visibility, convenience and proximity. You are more likely to eat something that is more visible (even if it's a photo on a menu), more convenient (something you can eat in five minutes as opposed to one you need to spend an hour preparing) and physically nearer to you (at eye level in the fridge as opposed to on the top shelf of the pantry).

As an example, let's use this knowledge to make yourself more likely to eat vegetables: you can keep them ready-cut (convenient), at eye level in the fridge (visible and nearer to you) and wrapped in clear plastic (visible). You could also use these environmental influences to help curb a candy habit you've developed at the office: stop walking by the vending machine during the day and don't keep any cash on you. Having to head all the way out to the car might make it just inconvenient enough to stop doing it, and you won't have the visual trigger of seeing the actual colorful candy bar wrappers.

Social Environment

Many of our choices are affected by the people we share our lives with, including our food behaviors and selections. The first success tactic I recommend is learning from a healthy example. There's a saying that "you are the composite of the five people you spend the most time with," and in terms of eating, it certainly has some truth to it. You're more likely to eat well and exercise if your friends do too. Spend time with people who overeat, emotionally eat or drink to excess and you are more likely to do the same. Likewise, spending more time with people who engage in healthy behaviors can rub off on you and teach you a thing or two. Consider if there's someone in your life with healthy habits that you might spend a bit more time around, ask some questions or just observe on the sly. Learn something from the people you know who have been practicing consistently healthy lifestyles for years.

Likewise, your eating habits affect those around you too. Luckily, getting lean doesn't mean sacrificing your friends, alienating your spouse or inconveniencing your coworkers. Garnering support from these parties will greatly increase your chances for permanent weight-loss success, but getting support from your friends and family isn't always as simple as telling them your plans. People who care about you are likely to subconsciously want you to stay the same (after all, they love you as is), so they may unknowingly voice subtle or not-so-subtle resistance to your intentions to change. Here are some communication strategies that can help you meet with less resistance and win the support of your family, coworkers and friends.

FOR MINIMAL RESISTANCE, EXPLAIN THE *WHY* FIRST, THEN THE *WHAT*.

It's common to start a conversation by telling someone first what we are going to change. Then, we hear their resistance to it, and respond with our reasons in effort to convince them. However, starting with the *reason for the change* is more likely to bring the other person along in sharing your mind-set and, if applicable, seeking the solution to a problem. Then you can mention the solution or change you have in mind and are likely to be met with less resistance to it.

Example (starting with why, then mention what): "I want to take better care of my health and set a good example for the kids. I know healthy dinners would help, so I'm planning on cooking more at home and getting takeout less for us all. Would you support me in that, and help make sure we've got groceries here for cooking at home?"

Example of what is *not* recommended (starting with the change or asking something of the other person): "Would you help me more with grocery shopping? I want to get takeout less often and cook more meals here, and I think it would be better for all of us." (It's likely that the person of whom this is being asked won't hear anything beyond the request for more work from them.)

STRATEGIES FOR FOOD PUSHERS

Especially at holiday time, family members can get pushy, encouraging you to eat more than you want to or indulge in items you politely passed on. While this can be highly stressful to the healthy eater, it generally isn't out of malice but out of love and a want to be accepted. Wanting you to have seconds of pie is another language for many mothers of wanting you to accept them and their love. Rather than risk bruised feelings by saying no over and over, you may ease the situation by acknowledging what the food pusher is really after. You might try, "I love you and I love your cooking, Mom, but I really don't need any more pie!" "I'll never have enough of your love, Aunt Daisy, but I don't have room left for any more of your cookies." Add a smile and a hug and they will likely let it go without hurt feelings.

Remember that hosts or family members generally want you to have a good time and be happy, and providing an abundance of food is one way of doing that. If you mention that you are "on a diet" or comment that you shouldn't eat any more "because you want to lose weight," I guarantee that you will get resisting commentary from your family or friends to try to change your mind. From their viewpoint, they see you (a person they are fond of) resisting an apparent pleasure (dessert) because you are unhappy with your current self. They will want to change that out of love for you! They will reassure you that you look fine, that you can have a little, that it won't kill you and so forth. They mean well, and their underlying intent isn't to sabotage your efforts to get healthier—they just want you to be happy, feel good and enjoy the moment.

My secret weapon against loved ones encouraging you to overeat is to *give a positive reason* when you decline additional servings of stuffing or say no to taking home leftover pie. "I've been eating less sugar lately, and I feel amazing!" is tough to contend with, because who would want you to feel less amazing? Other things to try are, "I sleep so much better when I'm not too full," and, "I'm at the perfect Goldilocks fullness now, so content but not uncomfortable. I'm staying here!"

Unfortunately, some food pushers aren't as benevolent as well-meaning family and friends. It's common among weight-conscious women in particular to encourage other women to eat indulgently as a way to mitigate their own guilt over what they are consuming. It can even get subtly competitive. In this instance, the food pusher isn't acting out of love or wanting acceptance, and they probably don't give a hoot if you're happy or not. They push high-calorie food on you to feel better about themselves or justify what they want to eat. It's unfortunately the case that having a partner in crime (or cake or ice cream consumption) makes it feel less damaging psychologically for a person to act in a way that defies their values. How you choose to respond may depend on the person and your relationship with them. The simplest strategy, appropriate for people you aren't close to, such as office coworkers passing out cake at an office party, is to politely decline and allow them to make their own decision without your involvement. If it's a friend proposing a social outing or something to share, you may suggest an alternate activity you can do so that you aren't losing out on time together. We generally don't recommend trying to change the other person's mind or talking them out of their indulgence, just keep your eyes on your own behavior, and bear in mind that food pushers' actions may have nothing to do with you and everything to do with their judgment of themselves.

WHAT TO DO

Physical Environment

Odds are, you make most of your food and eating decisions in four physical environments: your home kitchen, your workplace, restaurants and the grocery store.

Think about each location separately, and for each one:

- Ask yourself how you can make the healthier options more visible, more convenient or physically nearer to you. Write down your ideas.

- Next, consider how you can make unhealthy foods less visible, less convenient or physically inaccessible. Write these down too.

- Commit to making at least one change to your physical environment to support your healthy habits.

Social Environment

Consider the people in your life, and find someone who practices a consistently healthy lifestyle. Learn something from them by observing, or simply ask them how they do it.

Turn your accomplices into cheerleaders. Consider people in your social circle who have been accomplices; anybody who encouraged or joined you in your unhealthy behaviors. Turn them into cheerleaders by explaining your goals and requesting their support in your efforts to form new, healthy habits.

When speaking to your soon-to-be cheerleaders and family about your new habits, explain *why* you're making the change before talking about *what* will be different.

Last, don't let food pushers pressure you into eating anything you don't want to. Respond lovingly to keep relationships undamaged, or just politely decline. People who care about you want more than anything to see you happy and feeling good, so mentioning that your healthy behaviors contribute to feeling great is a great way to bring them on your side.

In your habit tracker, create a place to check off when you have completed each part of this assignment, making one change to your physical environment and one to your social environment. Aim to complete these as soon as you can, but within the next two weeks. After you have checked off each assignment, continue the habit of managing your environment by continually cultivating a helpful physical setup and supportive social network around you. You don't need to keep these two habit lines in your tracker, but if you notice down the road that your progress is slowing or that you have trouble maintaining your goal weight, revisiting this topic can be an integral part of resetting your habits.

HABIT	1	2	3	4	5	6	7	8	9	10	11	12	13	14
Eat 3 or 4 meals without snacking														
Hunger Mastery (hunger for 30–60 minutes before eating)														
Eat just enough at each meal														
Eat mostly (or all) whole foods														
Eat at least 6 cups of vegetables														
Reduce or eliminate liquid calories														
30–40 grams of protein at each meal														
15 grams of fat approx. at each meal														
Choose low-glycemic starches in small portions if extra carbohydrates are needed														
Follow intense exercise with a meal containing starchy carbohydrate, if applicable														

(continued)

HABIT	1	2	3	4	5	6	7	8	9	10	11	12	13	14
Keep track of treats (Goal for these 2 weeks: <25 total)														
Alchohol or caloric drinks (1 per drink)														
Sweets, desserts, candy (1 per cupcake, slice of cake, cookie, ounce of chocolate, ½ cup ice cream or frozen yogurt)														
Deep-fried food: chips, tortilla chips (1 per handful)														
Sugar added to coffee, tea, cereal or yogurt (1 per tsp)														
Processed foods (cereal bars, protein bars, ramen, etc.)														
Complete assignment: shape my physical environment														
Complete assignment: shape my social environment														

LEAN HABIT 14:
CONQUER EMOTIONAL EATING

I'm not saying you have a problem with emotional eating. But if you do, I'd like to help, since it's one of the most formidable barriers to achieving lasting weight loss. On a personal level, this is a topic close to my heart because my own life includes an epic journey to combat and eventually overcome my own emotional eating challenges—and I'm positive that if I can reform my habits (because I was in pretty deep!), you can too.

Emotional eating, defined as a tendency to eat in response to negative emotions, is correlated with BMI, waist circumference and body-fat percentage in both women and men. Evidence indicates that emotional eating accounts for at least some of the association between depression and weight gain, and the association of depression with increased snacking and consumption of sweet, energy-dense foods. In a sample of Dutch adults, emotional eating was a stronger predictor of a person becoming overweight than overeating in response to external food-related cues, such as the sight and smell of attractive food. Furthermore, evidence that emotional eating has dramatically increased among adults moved some obesity experts to propose, "Perhaps we should try to explain the current obesity epidemic from an emotion perspective."

Emotional eating has been shown to be particularly prevalent in obese adults, people with eating disorders and "restrained eaters" (frequent dieters or those who attempt to control their food intake as a means of body-weight control).

It's not clear exactly why some people eat in response to unpleasant emotions while others do not, but potential causes include the inability to differentiate between hunger and emotional distress; the desirability of food to distract from, numb or lessen an emotion; and the potential for eating to temporarily allow one to escape from a distressing state of self-awareness.

Avoiding all negative emotion isn't possible, but just because life's challenges aren't going anywhere doesn't mean that emotional eaters are stuck with maladaptive habits. Quite the opposite. Just as someone can adopt a new habit of eating more vegetables or going to the gym at any age, someone with the habit of eating in response to emotion can also change completely. A person's life doesn't have to become picture-perfect and idyllic for them to defeat emotional eating. After all, it's not the emotions that cause problems, but the way in which negative emotions are dealt with.

WHAT CONTRIBUTES TO EMOTIONAL EATING?
Inability to Separate Hunger and Emotion

Emotional eating isn't an instinct with which we are born; it is learned, possibly from a very young age. Children who spend greater amounts of time eating while watching TV or playing video games are more prone to becoming emotional eaters, likely because mindless eating is characterized by inattention to hunger and satiety cues. Over time, it is possible to have difficulty identifying these states accurately, as well as differentiating them from other aroused states, such as times of heightened emotion.

Sensations of hunger and satiety also blur when they are ignored in efforts to control calories and lose weight. Focusing on following diet programs, meal plans or counting calories all detract from a person's ability to tell when they are hungry, when they are satisfied and how these sensations feel different to experience than emotions. So, if you've been dieting for decades, it's completely understandable to have a harder time discerning emotional stimuli from physical signals like hunger. If you've been consistently practicing Hunger Mastery for a while, you have likely made immense progress in feeling and recognizing hunger—yet long-standing habits of eating in response to stress or sadness don't just vaporize on their own.

Emotional Suppression

Environmental factors such as culture, parental discipline, abuse or trauma can cause people at any age to learn to suppress their feelings as a coping strategy. The *Diagnostic and Statistical Manual of Mental Disorders 4* defines suppression as "a defense mechanism in which a person intentionally avoids thinking about disturbing problems, desires, feelings or experiences." Suppression of emotions is a type of emotional regulation. However, unlike adaptive methods of handling emotion, suppression is linked with unfavorable outcomes, such as increased tendency toward depression, anxiety and poor physical health. Emotional suppression is linked to earlier death as well as increased risk of cardiovascular disease, hypertension and cancer.

RESEARCH STUDIES HAVE SHOWN THAT PEOPLE WHO HABITUALLY SUPPRESS EMOTIONS EAT MORE DURING EMOTIONAL EXPERIENCES THAN THOSE WHO DO NOT, PARTICULARLY COMFORT FOODS HIGH IN FAT AND SUGAR.

Research studies have shown that people who habitually suppress emotions eat more during emotional experiences than those who do not, particularly comfort foods high in fat and sugar. Furthermore, people who are instructed by researchers to suppress emotions in an experimentally induced emotional state also increase food intake compared to those who are instructed to reappraise the stimulus or those who are given no instruction at all. Interestingly, the intensity of emotion makes no difference in whether someone turns to food or not. It's not how sad a person feels about a particular event that determines if they eat in response, it's what they do with the sadness.

Other Factors

Studies have found that emotional eating is more prevalent among people who employ rigid dietary restraint and dichotomous ("black or white") thinking. Alexithymia, difficulty with identifying and verbalizing emotions, is strongly correlated with emotional eating, disordered eating and obesity. It has been suggested that alexithymic people prefer to act rather than talk about their emotions, and eating can be a convenient and accessible way to act on emotion. Psychological inflexibility, the unwillingness to experience certain negative experiences, is also commonly associated with emotional eating as well as other maladaptive coping strategies.

WHAT CAN BE DONE

Separate Hunger and Emotion

One of the earliest habits in this system got you started on building your skills at sensing hunger. Hopefully, the weeks you spent tuning in to physiological hunger have gotten you more acquainted with what hunger feels like, and the specific nuances of how hunger is a different experience than an emotionally heightened state. Differentiating between the two is critical, and a necessary step in the process of learning to meet the actual need you are having at a given moment and not mistake it for another one.

If you still feel like you've got work to do in this area, though, don't worry. You've got time, and luckily every day provides several opportunities to tune in and feel hunger. Each day also provides a rich experience of different emotions, some of which may be gentle and some of which may be strong. I invite you to observe your emotions as they come and go just as you've been practicing observing and experiencing hunger. This is a powerful step in breaking a conditioned pattern of emotional suppression. Allow yourself to feel. Ask yourself during the day, "How am I feeling?" and try to use a word besides good, bad or fine. Are you excited, eager, content, bored, lonely or anxious? Can you sense little bit of two or three different feelings at the same time?

As you observe your emotions, you may find yourself wondering, "What do I *do* with this feeling?" There is no single answer, but there are several helpful practices that I share with my clients to develop a set of healthy emotional skills and break away from eating as an emotion-regulation strategy.

Just Feel It

For a moment, consider that you might not have to do anything at all. If you've lived for decades under the assumption that you should act when you get an unpleasant emotion to make it go away, this might be a shocking suggestion: you do not need to fix it. No harm comes from just allowing yourself to feel a feeling. You don't have to do a thing. Emotions are powerless to harm you. In fact, allowing yourself to welcome and feel the way you do might be the most expedient path to feeling better.

Taking a mind-set of acceptance and non-judgment can make this easier. That means not judging your emotional state as invalid, silly or wrong. It also means not trying to force it into a particular mold by analyzing or justifying it.

How many times have you believed that a feeling or thought you were having was silly, stupid, childish or just plain wrong? For example, it's easy to feel like it's wrong to be angry with someone we love, and to suppress it, deny it and put on a happy face when we actually are kind of steamed. However, anger is a natural and healthy thing to feel, and it can help us open our mouths and ask for different behavior in the future or an apology. Suppressing it in silence can lead to passive aggression or resentment that seethes under the surface. It's much healthier to let yourself feel it, observe it and decide what you want to do, rather than denying that your anger exists. Even saying, "I notice I'm feeling angry," is a great place to start!

Note that allowing yourself to feel your emotions doesn't mean wallowing or clinging to them. It is quite possible to make yourself feel worse if you stew over a negative emotional experience, replay it in your mind like a video or retell the story to 30 other people (effectively reliving it yourself). Thinking a lot about your emotion, reinforcing it with "should" statements, labeling people or behaviors as "right" or "wrong" may all prolong and heighten your experience of feeling lousy. Instead, consider just observing the way you feel, acknowledging it as valid and going on with your day. If it stays with you, fine, but if it vaporizes, that's fine too. Typically, letting yourself freely feel something makes it lighter immediately and over hours and days it may ebb and flow again or just drift off completely.

Learn to Reappraise Instead of Suppress

I mentioned in an earlier section how suppressing one's feelings is a self-protective way to deal with them, but that it is associated with many negative outcomes, just one of which is an increased likelihood of engaging in emotional eating. Other types of emotional regulation, such as reappraisal, lead to healthier outcomes than suppression. Reappraisal means changing the way you think about an emotional situation to alter its emotional impact. For example, you can reappraise an unforeseen work obstacle as a chance to show your work ethic, thus lessening the frustration and negative feelings you experience. People who predominantly use suppression to regulate their emotions have been shown to increase food intake in an emotional state, while those who use cognitive reappraisal are less prone to emotional eating.

To try this one out, try to think of stimuli that bother you in a new way. I'm not saying lie to yourself; think of framing it in a way that is still true but less upsetting. You may have neglected to see the positive elements of some change, such as, "Although this was my second-choice position, it is a shorter commute and the benefits are equally good." You may also be able to reappraise a disappointment by revising your expectations. If you have unfairly rigid expectations of yourself (such as perfection) that lead to you being chronically disappointed, reappraising your imperfections can help you see them as human and harmless, not the end of the world. "I made two typos on a 94-page document, that's better than most people could do, and I did a thorough job. That's why we have an editor anyway."

While the topic may seem tangential for a weight-loss program, I've learned how incredibly beneficial it is with my personal coaching clients to help them develop healthy, realistic expectations of themselves, other people and the world. It leads to a lot less disappointment, strife and frustration in life. Lower levels of those feelings sure make it easier to consistently practice healthy habits too!

Strengthen Distress Tolerance

Many people who have struggled with emotional eating or other maladaptive coping skills have a sense of urgency when they get upset. They want to flee or do something drastic to change the situation **now**. Building resilience helps a person trust that they can manage uncomfortable sensations (emotional or physical) and be less upset by them.

You don't have to go out of your way to create discomfort solely for this purpose, just bear in mind that when life hands you the inevitable challenge, it is an opportunity to prove and strengthen your resilience. You can handle it. It might not be easy, it might not be fun, but you can do hard things.

Whether you are in physical discomfort or emotional pain, one powerful strategy to get through it calmly is to become totally present. To do that, you'll tune in to the current moment only. Situations which *feel* intolerable or excruciating are often so distressing because we are getting ahead of ourselves with worry or fear about the future, when right this moment actually isn't so bad. In this very moment, there is often no problem at all; it's dipping into the past to feel regret or shame or anger that heightens our suffering, or venturing ahead into the future that causes us worry or fear. When you find yourself feeling upset or even just a little uneasy, come back to this very moment.

Practice Flexible Dietary Restraint

Rigid dietary control is associated with increased emotional eating, binge eating and disinhibition (overeating). On the other hand, flexible dietary restraint is correlated with lower BMI and greater success with long-term weight maintenance. Rigid control is characterized by all-or-nothing thinking, forbidding certain foods, calorie counting and meal skipping. Flexible dietary control is characterized by moderating the frequency and portion of certain foods, enjoying a variety of foods and allowing your calorie intake to vary naturally from day to day.

WHERE TO START

Early habits you learned in this book have given you a head start in building the skills necessary for ending emotional eating. Hunger Mastery has helped you become more familiar with true hunger and how it is a different sensation from what emotions feel like. Observing your treats intake and allowing for your favorite foods in appropriate quantities is a form of flexibly controlling your intake without rigid abstinence.

What I'll ask you to do next that *is* new is to **practice sensing your emotions, accepting them and letting yourself feel them.** Doing this for just a moment before each time you eat means at least three practice sessions a day are automatically built in to your life, but the benefits only increase if you do it more often, so feel free to practice it anytime. Especially if you get a sudden overwhelming urge to inhale a whole row of Oreos, it's a great time to check in and ask yourself what you're feeling.

I spotted this note posted in our client forum recently which shows what a game-changer this habit can be:

"I'm sure I'm not the only person in here who has previously eaten her feelings away when they are of the uncomfortable variety. Just as an FYI, yesterday I had extreme emotional discomfort—like, completely labile and on the edge of tears and just feeling like a miserable human over something(s) very trivial, but still, feelings aren't logical sometimes.

For the first time I can remember, I didn't do anything to distract myself from the discomfort. I didn't eat, I didn't read, I didn't watch TV, I didn't get on the computer. I just sat and FELT. It was very, very, VERY uncomfortable. I went to work, still on the verge of tears, sure I was going to be a basket case all day.

But you know what? They just …WENT AWAY. I didn't have to DO anything to make that happen. I'm not sure where I read it, but I know somewhere Georgie said something to the effect that you don't have to do anything when you have a bad feeling, you can just quietly sit there and experience it. Like hunger, it won't kill you to have it.

And she's right. Georgie Fear, you're freakin' brilliant. Thanks."

Update your habit tracker with your next daily habit to practice: "Allow, accept and feel my emotions before each meal (and as needed)."

HABIT	1	2	3	4	5	6	7	8	9	10	11	12	13	14
Eat 3 or 4 meals without snacking														
Hunger Mastery (hunger for 30–60 minutes before eating)														
Eat just enough at each meal														
Eat mostly (or all) whole foods														
Eat at least 6 cups of vegetables														
Reduce or eliminate liquid calories														
30–40 grams of protein at each meal														
15 grams of fat approx. at each meal														
Choose low-glycemic starches in small portions if extra carbohydrates are needed														
Follow intense exercise with a meal containing starchy carbohydrate, if applicable														
Keep track of treats (Goal for these 2 weeks: <25 total)														
Alchohol or caloric drinks (1 per drink)														
Sweets, desserts, candy (1 per cupcake, slice of cake, cookie, ounce of chocolate, ½ cup ice cream or frozen yogurt)														
Deep-fried food: chips, tortilla chips (1 per handful)														
Sugar added to coffee, tea, cereal or yogurt (1 per tsp)														
Processed foods (cereal bars, protein bars, ramen, etc.)														
Complete assignment: shape my physical environment														
Complete assignment: shape my social environment														
Allow, accept and feel my emotions (before each meal + as needed)														

WHERE YOU CAN GO NEXT

As you can tell from this chapter, there are many steps and skills to be acquired in beating emotional eating. The "assigned habit" of learning to identify, allow and accept your emotions is a great step to start with, and you may find it creates a ripple effect of other positive changes in your emotional wellness.

Among the payoffs that follow, you may find yourself relieved to finally have *options* for what to do when you have strong emotions. They are not in control of you; you are choosing your response. You can choose to take no outward action and just experience your feelings (knowing that they are harmless and temporary), or there may be an appropriate response such as speaking up if you disagree, getting water if you're thirsty, apologizing if you've wronged someone or just getting out of the house and taking a walk in the fresh air if you're restless. Regardless of whether you choose to take action or not, you'll be leagues ahead of the days when you denied the emotion existed at all or tried to stuff it down or numb it with food.

A BIT OF MY STORY

Had there been a competition, I would have won titles for emotional suppression not too long ago. Any negative emotions that I didn't suppress I immediately tried to escape. I used obsessive dieting and compulsive exercise to escape sometimes, and at other times I just ate lots and lots of cookies. Emotional overeating and undereating are two heads on the same beast for many people; they may seem like opposites, but both are efforts to manipulate or control your emotional state through food. I made it almost three decades on this planet without allowing myself to feel anger, to disagree with anyone I loved or to speak my mind if there was the slightest chance of being met with disapproval. I didn't rock the boat, but sometimes I tried to eat my way out of it.

In other words, I know how easy it to not even know you are suppressing things. I had no clue. I thought I was just a really nice, accommodating person! No one else will tell you (because they can't know) that you are suppressing your feelings all day long. And they sure won't complain about how easy you are to get along with. I might never have changed if my health hadn't fallen apart. What started as a curious tendency toward getting queasy became a clear pattern: difficult conversations were immediately followed by bouts of nausea. When I agreed to go somewhere I didn't want to, I got nauseous. When I got blamed for things unfairly, I got nauseated. When someone made an insensitive or racist comment, the nausea would almost bring me to the ground. As much as I didn't like it, I saw what it was. It was making me sick to deny the fact that I had an opinion, and if I never let my own feelings appear on my decision-making radar it would never change. I spent thousands of dollars on medical treatments trying to cure a problem that I was actually causing.

The best thing about learning you are the cause of all your own problems is that you hold the key to fixing them all. After you stop kicking yourself, I have found, it's quite empowering. I started with the very habit assignment I gave you in this chapter, that three times a day I would ask myself what I was feeling. It was slow going at first, like trying to speak a language in which you know only a dozen words, but I got better at it the more I practiced. From there, changes in my life started to unfold naturally (and the nausea finally went away). I hope for you the process also flows; as you gather positive momentum, you feel better and better, and food becomes just food, not a coping mechanism.

Once you let yourself feel your feelings, the next step is to honor them. Speak up, express yourself, defend yourself, take care of your own needs and say no if you are too tired or overextended to accept a commitment. While this can feel risky or scary the first few times, tune in to the outcomes and you'll see: no one minds. You won't become a social outcast; in fact, you may earn more respect for expressing your authentic self. People will often approve of you more when you stop fearing their disapproval and just relax.

Discovering that the world actually accepts you as your authentic self is comforting beyond words. Suddenly, dozens of cookies did not have to give their lives to get me through the week. I felt more at ease, less anxious and, surprisingly, considerably less obsessed with controlling my weight or food intake. Saying no once in a while diffused my undercurrent of resentment and martyrdom. If you've ever been halfway through a pint of ice cream and found yourself wishing others could see how hard your life is (like the camera atop the helmet of a snowboarder) because *then they would understand*, you might benefit from saying no a bit more. No one is watching. No one is giving you points for making yourself suffer. Shoving food in our mouths while we're standing at the sink after a hard day or week is an ineffective way of flipping the bird to the world for how cruel it's being to us.

Kicking emotional eating is hard, but the dividends it pays off are far reaching and don't stop at a leaner physique.

LEAN HABIT 15:
HYDRATION POWER

"Drink more water" is a piece of advice you've probably heard a thousand times. I understand that improving your hydration probably isn't the most thrilling and exciting habit in which to invest your energy. But it is absolutely worthwhile, even if it is the oldest advice in the book for shedding pounds.

WHAT TO DO

To be fully hydrated, adults need about one to one and a half milliliters of fluid for every calorie burned, which means that most people require about two liters (2,000 milliliters or 64 ounces) of fluid each day. For your next habit, **practice making sure to drink at least two liters, or 64 ounces, of fluid a day.** As covered earlier in this book, liquid calories should be minimized, but calorie-free drinks can help you meet your fluid needs just fine. Don't worry if your beverages contain caffeine, since caffeinated and non-caffeinated fluids hydrate the body equally well. So if coffee or tea is part of your daily beverage intake, you can count those two toward your 64 ounces.

Research indicates that people consume 75 to 89 percent of their fluids with meals, with relatively little fluid consumption between meals. Studies have also shown that proximity helps with increasing water intake; having water available on your desk or dining table greatly increases the amount of water you drink, compared to having to walk 20 feet to obtain a drink. So to get up to 64 ounces of fluid per day, remember to keep your beverages easy to access. You can fill a water bottle and keep it on your desk within reach, brew a cup of tea before a daily office meeting and place a pitcher of water on the table for family meals. You can also help form a habit by anchoring your intake to other things you do each day, for example, drinking a glass of water when you wake up, hitting the water fountain between exercises at the gym (figure an ounce per swallow) or always polishing off a bottle of water before you pick up the kids from school or after you walk the dog.

Tip: if getting up at night to urinate becomes inconvenient, front-load your water earlier in the day so you don't need to drink lots in the hours before bedtime and you sleep more soundly.

WHY IT'S WORTH IT

In an analysis of three large-scale cohort studies involving more than 120,000 people, water intake was shown to be associated with less weight gain over time. Specifically, for each additional cup of water consumed, a person could be expected to gain 0.13 kilogram less weight over four years. If the cup of water replaced a sugar-sweetened beverage or glass of juice, the effect rose to 0.49 kilogram less weight gain.

Epidemiological evidence suggests that water drinkers consume an average of 194 fewer calories per day than non–water drinkers, which amounts to 9 percent lower total calorie intake.

HOW IT WORKS

Does water make you burn more calories? Maybe. Water might induce a thermogenic response and temporarily increase metabolic rate. While some studies have observed a considerable metabolic rate increase after drinking water, other studies have found no effect. So the jury is out, but there's a chance it helps you burn a few more calories to drink up, especially if the water is cold and your body has to do some work to heat it up to body temperature. One thing we know for sure it won't do is hurt you.

The effect of water to keep weight gain at bay is more likely due to altered food behaviors. Water can help fill you up or take the edge off hunger. Drinking water before or with a meal has been shown to reduce subjects' ratings of hunger and increase perceived fullness, but it's not clear whether free-living people actually eat less as a result of drinking it with meals. Some trials have shown that drinking water before meals results in less food intake, but similar studies have found no effect. Some evidence shows that eating foods with a high fluid content such as fresh fruits and vegetables has a greater impact on reducing subsequent food intake than drinking water as a beverage. (Just in case you needed another reminder that fresh fruits and vegetables are good things to include at mealtime.) It's tough to say whether drinking more water is, by itself, impactful enough to reduce someone's calorie intake and produce weight loss. However, evidence does seem to indicate that it helps people stick to and get better results from a weight-loss program.

Weight-loss-intervention studies suggest that subjects lose more weight when additional water intake is prescribed along with a hypocaloric diet. In a 12-week weight-loss program, one group of subjects was instructed to drink a 16-ounce bottle of water before each meal, while the other group received no instructions on water intake. Over the 12-week study, the water group lost 44 percent more weight, a difference of about four pounds (two kilograms).

In addition to possibly helping augment fullness from lower-calorie meals, drinking enough water can also aid weight loss by paring out eating occasions that aren't needed. Many people respond to thirst by reaching for food when, physiologically, they really need hydration. It's easy to do! Over time, the sensations of hunger and thirst can blur and a habit of eating in response to thirst can contribute to weight gain.

In the last lesson, we reviewed the importance of being able to differentiate emotion from hunger; here we'll point out that separating thirst from hunger is another valuable skill to getting and staying lean for life.

One of the early signs of dehydration is fatigue. Before you feel thirsty, you may notice being tired or mentally less sharp. Eating in response to fatigue is a common behavior resulting in extra calorie intake. So staying well hydrated can help keep you alert while avoiding a common dietary stumbling block.

Update your habit tracker and start logging your practice with staying hydrated.

HABIT	1	2	3	4	5	6	7	8	9	10	11	12	13	14
Eat 3 or 4 meals without snacking														
Hunger Mastery (hunger for 30—60 minutes before eating)														
Eat just enough at each meal														
Eat mostly (or all) whole foods														
Eat at least 6 cups of vegetables														
Reduce or eliminate liquid calories														
30–40 grams of protein at each meal														
15 grams of fat approx. at each meal														
Choose low-glycemic starches in small portions if extra carbohydrates are needed														
Follow intense exercise with a meal containing starchy carbohydrate, if applicable														
Keep track of treats (Goal for these 2 weeks: <25 total)														
Alchohol or caloric drinks (1 per drink)														
Sweets, desserts, candy (1 per cupcake, slice of cake, cookie, ounce of chocolate, ½ cup ice cream or frozen yogurt)														
Deep-fried food: chips, tortilla chips (1 per handful)														
Sugar added to coffee, tea, cereal or yogurt (1 per tsp)														
Processed foods (cereal bars, protein bars, ramen, etc.)														
Complete assignment: shape my physical environment														
Complete assignment: shape my social environment														
Allow, accept and feel my emotions (before each meal + as needed)														
Stay hydrated (drink 64 oz today)														

LEAN HABIT 16:
GET ENOUGH SLEEP

WHAT TO DO

"It's not just about rest; sleep keeps your appetite calibrated."

Make getting seven hours of sleep a night your goal. If you need to set a bedtime, do it. Re-prioritizing your evening tasks to include less television time and more pillow time can go a long way to getting the sleep you need. If you've scheduled enough hours in bed but can't seem to fall or stay asleep for most of them, try the tips below, courtesy of the National Sleep Foundation.

NATIONAL SLEEP FOUNDATION ADVICE FOR GOOD SLEEP

If you have trouble sleeping, try the following tips:

• Treat your bedroom as your sanctuary from the stresses of the day. Create a comfortable sleeping environment, with a quality mattress and pillows, that is free of distractions.

• Be sure your bedroom is dark when you go to bed and will stay dark until you get the sleep you need. Use light-blocking curtains or shades to be sure your room stays dark.

• Establish a relaxing bedtime routine. Allow enough time to wind down and relax before going to bed.

• If you find yourself still lying awake after 20 minutes, get out of bed. Get up and do something relaxing in dim light until you are sleepy.

- Avoid exposure to bright light late at night. Dim your lights when it's close to bedtime, and use night lights for nighttime awakenings.

- Exercise regularly. Exercise in the morning can help you get the light exposure you need to set your biological clock. Avoid vigorous exercise close to bedtime if you are having problems sleeping.

- Use a sound conditioner or earplugs to block unwanted sounds.

- Avoid caffeinated beverages, large meals and alcohol right before bedtime.

- No late-afternoon or evening naps, unless you work nights. If you must nap, keep it under 45 minutes and before 3 p.m.

WHY IT'S WORTH IT

Not getting enough sleep is an independent risk factor for obesity and many other health conditions. Epidemiological studies reveal that getting fewer than seven hours of sleep is associated with current and future development of obesity. In other words, even if you are at a healthy weight today, you predispose yourself to future weight gain by shortchanging yourself on sleep! In research studies, insufficient sleep has been shown to increase energy intake, especially in the evenings after dinner, and lead to weight gain in as little as five days. Furthermore, transitioning to an adequate sleep pattern has been shown to result in decreased energy intake from fat and carbohydrates, and weight loss. So not only would you have better energy during the day (and fewer under-eye circles to conceal), but hitting the pillow earlier makes it easier to eat less and get slimmer. That's not something we tend to think of when we're halfheartedly telling ourselves, "Yeah, I should be turning in soon ... after one more show."

HOW IT WORKS

Not getting enough shut-eye dials up a person's appetite by increasing amounts of the hunger-stimulating hormone ghrelin and decreasing levels of the appetite-suppressing hormone leptin. (Remember that leptin is a hormone that communicates information regarding the body's energy balance to the brain.) In experimental conditions, restricting sleep to four hours a night produces markedly lower levels of circulating leptin than when subjects are adequately rested, despite similar calorie intake, physical activity and stable BMI. Decreases in thyroid-stimulating hormone (TSH) and impaired insulin sensitivity have also been reported when sleep was limited to four hours per night. That makes sleep-deprived people hungrier and less likely to feel like moving around during the day, meaning they burn fewer overall calories than if they had gotten seven hours of rest.

SO JUST HOW MUCH HUNGRIER ARE WE TALKING?

You may have felt firsthand (perhaps during the last diet you were on) how being in a large calorie deficit makes you feel very hungry. It's not in your imagination; research subjects experience it too. Subjects on hypocaloric diets consistently report increased hunger and desire to eat, and the effect is correlated with the magnitude of the calorie deficit. One of the biological mechanisms at work is decreased leptin activity in the hypothalamus. Leptin decrease also contributes to the decrease in resting metabolism seen after weight loss.

Since I'm interested in teaching you how to lose fat as comfortably as possible, I definitely don't want your leptin levels dropping due to shortened sleep. To help give some perspective of the impact of sleep on leptin, bear in mind that a caloric deficit of 900 per day has been shown to cause a 22 percent drop in leptin in lean, healthy volunteers. (That's a big deficit; it means eating only about half of what average adults need to main their weight.) So eating half of your calorie needs causes a 22 percent drop in leptin, which makes you hungry as a bear, got it?

Let's compare that to what happens when you under-sleep. In a study published in 2004 in the *Journal of Clinical Endocrinology & Metabolism*, six days of four-hour sleep restriction produced a 26 percent reduction in peak leptin levels compared to allowing up to 12 hours in bed. A study published in the *International Journal of Endocrinology* in 2012 reports a 19 percent decrease in leptin concentration after five consecutive nights of five-hour sleep limitation. So, at least in the context of leptin, limiting yourself to four or five hours of sleep is like opting into the amount of extra hunger you'd feel if you had undereaten by 900 calories! Who needs extra hunger added to their life when trying to lose fat? I'm going to guess, not you.

Brain imaging studies have revealed that decreased sleep duration even makes your brain react differently to seeing food or images of food. Compared to when they were well rested after nine hours in bed, subjects who were roused after only four hours showed heightened brain reactivity to food stimuli. Areas of the brain linked to motivation, reward-seeking and desire were more activated by food images when people were tired, suggesting that sleep deprivation leaves people more susceptible to food temptation and overeating than they are when getting more sleep. Personally, I've never had my brain scanned, but my experience has been exactly that: it feels considerably tougher to resist edible temptations after even one night of too-little rest. String several nights together and the effect gets even worse.

So here's what your habit tracker should look like with this habit:

HABIT	1	2	3	4	5	6	7	8	9	10	11	12	13	14
Hunger Mastery (hunger for 30–60 minutes before eating)														
Eat just enough at each meal														
Eat mostly (or all) whole foods														
Eat at least 6 cups of vegetables														
Reduce or eliminate liquid calories														
30–40 grams of protein at each meal														
15 grams of fat approx. at each meal														
Choose low-glycemic starches in small portions if extra carbohydrates are needed														
Follow intense exercise with a meal containing starchy carbohydrate, if applicable														

HABIT									9	10	11	12	13	14
Keep track of treats (Goal for these 2 weeks: <25 total)														
Alchohol or caloric drinks (1 per drink)														
Sweets, desserts, candy (1 per cupcake, slice of cake, cookie, ounce of chocolate, ½ cup ice cream or frozen yogurt)														
Deep-fried food: chips, tortilla chips (1 per handful)														
Sugar added to coffee, tea, cereal or yogurt (1 per tsp)														
Processed foods (cereal bars, protein bars, ramen, etc.)														
Complete assignment: shape my physical environment														
Complete assignment: shape my social environment														
Allow, accept and feel my emotions (before each meal + as needed)														
Stay hydrated (drink 64 oz today)														
Get at least 7 hours of sleep														

TROUBLESHOOTING

At this point we've covered the most common and important habits that I use with clients, and you've gotten all the essential information on the core habits that just about everyone works on. Additional individualized habits often help people on their way to weight-loss success, such as reducing and managing stress, systematizing food shopping and preparation, letting go of ineffective behaviors like calorie counting or restricting or forming new routines to get through the times of day when you feel especially frazzled. For complete personalization, you can enroll in our coaching program and have an expert coach help tailor your habits to your life and your goals.

If you have been completing all the habits consistently each day, you should be seeing fat-loss results already. Anywhere from one-half to one pound a week is a typical rate of loss for my clients. Some weeks you may lose more, some weeks less, but over time it should average out to one-half to one pound each week. In the upcoming section I'll go through what to do if your weight loss stalls, slows or never really gets started.

TROUBLESHOOT 1: I'M DOING ALL THE HABITS BUT THE SCALE ISN'T MOVING

If you aren't losing weight, you need to create an additional calorie deficit by eating less. Three habits that are most helpful to revisit and tune up are Hunger Mastery, Eating Just Enough and your treat budget.

Hunger Mastery: You may be mistaking other internal sensations for hunger, or may be failing to distinguish between a desire to eat and hunger. To brush up on your Hunger Mastery, verify that you are experiencing true, belly-centered hunger before each meal, and jot down the time when you begin to experience hunger to make sure you aren't just "checking the box" on experiencing it and are actually having it for the full 30 to 60 minutes. If you are aiming for 30 minutes each time and want better results, go to 60 minutes of experiencing hunger before you eat.

You can also observe how many times each week you ate without being hungry for 30 to 60 minutes before (the blanks in your tracker with no *x*) and aim to reduce those instances. See what's getting in your way those times; did you overestimate how much you needed to eat at lunch and didn't have an appetite for dinner? Maybe you had social plans to eat at a certain time with friends. You might have let stress from your job lure you into snacking on candy, or an emotional upset could have sent you heading for food to cope. Whatever it is, look for what you can do make it easier to adhere to your habit even in that circumstance. That might mean paring back lunch on days you have early dinner plans or brainstorming alternates for diffusing stress and coping with emotions.

Eating Just Enough: To keep your skills sharp on this habit and keep progress going, you may need to redefine what feels like just enough, possibly several times. If what you are currently eating feels perfectly comfortable and you are maintaining your weight but want to lose, eat just a little less. You may have to let yourself be slightly more uncomfortable for short periods of time. You won't suffer unbearable agony from three bites less, and that small change could get your weight loss going. It will feel a little different at first, but soon that new amount will feel like your new normal.

Notice any incidents in which you think you ate more than you needed to. You might have justified eating more than normal because it was a holiday or special occasion, or you might have simply gotten so into the excellent taste of a meal that you didn't notice you were satisfied. Both are common and very easy to do. You can help yourself succeed by reminding yourself that you don't have to be perfect, and it's okay to choose to get more full sometimes, but it does all count. Even if it is someone's birthday or a holiday, everything you eat still counts when it comes to weight loss. Remember to eat slowly, especially when you eat out or enjoy extra-tasty food, so you don't mistakenly bypass your satisfaction point.

Treats Budget: Ensure that you are counting *everything* in those categories, and not forgetting anything. Even if it's one bite, mark it down as a decimal, but don't ignore it. If you aren't losing weight, try reducing the number of treats you have per week and really savoring the ones you have. If your sweet tooth is tripping you up by leading to high sugar intake, try having fruit instead, chewing a piece of gum after meals or having a cup of tea with no-calorie sweetener.

TROUBLESHOOT 2: I WAS NAILING THINGS AT FIRST BUT THEN STARTED SLIPPING AS I ADDED MORE HABITS

It takes repeated practice to change habits, and you may need more time to really cement a new habit before adding a new skill on top. Beware the common trap of continually seeking more information, when what you need most is to practice application of what you know. It's easy to get bogged down in reading tons of fitness and nutrition articles, but once you've got the essential information on a change you want to make, you need to practice it, not just bounce on to the next topic.

If a particular habit feels challenging to do each day even after two weeks, you are not ready to add another one. Practice the first habit until it becomes very easy, almost automatic, and only then add the second habit. Give the second habit as much practice as you need, until it too requires very little thinking, before adding in the third habit. Until it's easy, keep practicing. If you've gotten to the point where you have lots of habits but you're only kinda-sorta doing them, pare back. Simplify to one habit and nail it. Then, go slowly as you add others.

TROUBLESHOOT 3: I SKIPPED OR MODIFIED THE HABITS AND I'M NOT LOSING WEIGHT

If you bypassed certain habits, you might have needed those habits more than you believed at first glance. I suggest reviewing the whole list, and even if it seems like certain things don't apply to you, give them a try for two weeks to double-check. What do you have to lose? You might find out that you eat fewer vegetables, more treats and more liquid calories than you thought. Or you may have never thought your emotions had anything to do with your food intake, but a little attention to allowing and accepting your feelings could have positive effects for reining in a mysteriously ferocious appetite. To give yourself the best chance at success, you'll want to do all of the habits.

If you scaled habits downward to create a more manageable level of challenge, I applaud you. But be careful that you didn't scale habits to accommodate the way you already do things so you didn't have to change. If you scaled the liquid calories habit to say, "No liquid calories except my daily coffee with cream," and didn't end up modifying anything because those are the only liquid calories you drink, then you haven't reduced your liquid calories at all. You have to change something to get results, so even if you feel very protective of the status quo, try to be open to changing, at least as a temporary, conditional experiment. If you absolutely hate the new routine, you can always go back to the old one. But you just might discover that the change you resisted so persistently wasn't as bad as you thought.

TROUBLESHOOT 4: I KNOW WHAT TO DO BUT I DON'T DO IT CONSISTENTLY. WHAT'S WRONG WITH ME?!

Nothing is wrong with you, but your thinking could probably benefit from some redirecting. If you are frequently struggling to practice your habits, or finding yourself making excuses to not do them today, you're not sunk! Let me help you out by explaining a quick (and simplified) version of behavior motivation:

The way you think determines how you feel, and the way you feel determines how you act.

Emotion is a far more powerful driver of behavior than knowledge. Thinking about your own life experience, you probably can come up with several examples of times when emotions were much more powerful than facts in governing your behavior. Even if you know something is safe (such as flying or being hungry), if you're afraid of it, you are highly likely to make efforts to avoid it. Even if you know wearing high heels isn't great for your posture, dang it, if you feel sexy and incredibly confident in heels, at least from time to time you're going to put them on anyway. Feelings are powerful, so when you want to mold your behaviors to sculpt a leaner, healthier body, you need your emotions to be on your side, not just knowledge. Negative emotions about the behaviors you are trying to cement will poison your motivation to do them.

If you start to feel deprived or rebellious, think about what you are choosing, not what you are turning down. Every choice in life means letting one option go. We are always saying yes to one thing and no to another. Focusing on what you are saying *yes* to keeps your mind-set positive and reminds you that you are in the driver's seat. Thinking that you "have to" eat vegetables or "can't" eat a dessert is not true. No one is taking anything away from you or forcing you to adopt these habits. If you've read this far, odds are you want to make a change for the healthier. Remind yourself as often as needed that you do not *have* to do this, you *want* to do this.

If you are hesitant to make a change because you think about how much you enjoy the food you'd be giving up or having less of (your afternoon snack or beers on Saturday, for example), ask yourself if keeping your current behavior is worth more to you than a leaner body, and give yourself the option to choose either. It really is 100 percent up to you.

Remember that predictions about a potential change are often more dramatic and negative than the change actually is. You might find that once you actually try the change, it won't be nearly as bad as you thought it would be. For extra mental leverage, I remind clients that they can think of getting leaner and healthier as an experiment or trial run. If you do find that having the leaner body is not worth what you had to change to get it, you could go back to some or all of the old way of doing things. Try to remain open to the idea that making any one change isn't all that hard, especially after you get used to it, and give yourself time to find ways to make it easy and pleasant.

TROUBLESHOOT 5: TRYING TO FORM HABITS WHILE COUNTING CALORIES

Trying to stick to a calorie budget and trying to use hunger and satiety to guide your eating simultaneously is a recipe for failure. You cannot build trust in something (your body and mind) while keeping it under constant scrutiny and surveillance. Counting calories enhances the perceived value of food (giving you stronger cravings and desire to eat), creates emotional stress, takes up a lot of your time and is a huge distraction from the things which actually help you lose weight and keep it off: sensing how much you truly need to eat, learning how much is enough and knowing when you are hungry. When logging everything they eat, a person tends to develop a constant sense of wanting more food, but being leashed, not able to eat it freely. The limitation and scarcity mind-set creates more wanting, which creates more tension. I have never met a single person who liked counting calories. All the people I know (including myself) did it with a sense of anxiety, distrust of their own bodies and fear. It becomes a daily battle against the numbers, in which you lose all sight of feeling hunger, fullness and enjoyment of eating. This might be familiar to you if you have tried using calorie counting to lose weight before. It doesn't take too long of plugging your food into MyFitnessPal before you start to feel dependent on it. If you can't get to the Internet or use the app on your phone, you begin to feel like you don't know if you can eat or not! Vacations and eating out are far from relaxing; they can be a source of dread. While it can feel like keeping track of calories is helpful, and it often gives a comforting (false) sense of control, it prevents tuning in to your own body's signals, which you need to be able to do if you are going to eat for yourself. I take it you do not want to be 85 years old and still dependent on a phone app to tell you if you can drink your Ensure or not.

As a strategy to lose weight, my recommendation is to not count calories for an extended period, ever.

However, as an awareness-increasing exercise, completing a food log for a short interval can be a valuable snapshot to help troubleshoot your habits if you hit a plateau and aren't sure what's the problem. Objective data can shed light on a dietary stumbling block you may not even know exists, and bring to your attention a habit you might need to tune up. If you aren't sure why you aren't losing weight, performing an accurate calorie count can help clarify why you aren't in a calorie deficit. Your metabolism isn't broken, you are simply not in a calorie deficit, and counting up exactly how many calories you are eating for a few days can show you why.

Before you jump into putting a calorie tracking app on your phone or registering with a food logging website, consider the following:

Get Your Head in the Right Spot

If you want to know for sure where your calories are coming from, you have to be as accurate as possible with weighing and measuring all of your food. If you are not willing to do an honest, detailed and accurate inventory of absolutely everything you eat for several days, you are better off not doing one at all. Even rounded tablespoons instead of level tablespoons can throw off the numbers considerably. Estimating your portions will make your data completely unreliable. People who estimate their portion sizes in food diaries tend to produce food journals that confirm their existing beliefs. For example, a person who suspects that they have an abnormally slow metabolism, a condition which the science community has repeatedly shown to be almost always nonexistent, is likely to produce a food diary that represents only 50 percent of their true calorie intake. Some of this inaccuracy is introduced by estimating portions instead of measuring carefully, some of it from forgetting to include certain foods, beverages or condiments and some of it comes from popping bites of food into one's mouth while cooking and not realizing it. Do your best to not fall prey to your own bias; be as accurate and ruthless as possible, letting no bite escape your data collection.

Get Your Data Without Judging It

If you are committed to doing it accurately and fully, do a record of three to seven days but no more. Include at least one weekend day. If the program you are using involves selecting each food item from a database, be sure to choose entries which are as accurate as possible, preferably ones which have been validated by the USDA nutrient database. In addition to validated entries, many databases contain user-entered items which are not accurate. I encourage you to not get into analyzing or judging the data at all until you have finished collecting it. Leave that for after. Your job while doing a calorie count is to do it accurately for three to seven days and then stop.

Analyze Your Data and Adjust Your Habits

Once you have the data, remember that you want to use it to improve your habits in daily practice. Maintain a mind-set that you are looking for something you weren't aware of, so you can correct it, not trying to prove to the world that you are unfairly exempted from the laws of thermodynamics. Seek out the places you might be taking in extra calories with an open mind and interest in finding them.

Here are some things you might see in your data, and the corresponding habit to revisit to improve:

- If you are eating between-meal snacks, popping food into your mouth while cooking or doing excessive tasting, refocus on practicing eating three or four meals a day without eating in between.

- If you notice that some or many of your meals tend to be higher than 600 calories each, check the quantity of fruits and vegetables you are getting with each and see if you can bump it up. Usually, if a client is getting 300 to 450 grams of vegetables and fruits with every meal (2 to 3 cups, or 10 to 16 ounces), they naturally take in fewer calories to get satisfied. Meals with less than 300 grams of fresh veggies and fruit tend to be the higher calorie ones.

- If you notice that some of your meals are greater than 600 calories, ask yourself if you are truly eating "just enough" or if you are consuming more than you need to and could try a few bites less. Do not interpret the prior sentence as any implication that you are doing something wrong by eating 600 calories or more at a time. It is simply an invitation to double-check. You might need 600-calorie (or larger) meals, especially if you are active and have a high-calorie output. However, if you are not losing weight, you are fully meeting your energy needs and should be able to comfortably shave off three bites somewhere to create a small deficit without introducing significant physical discomfort.

- If you are falling below 30 grams of protein per meal, revisit the protein habit.

- If you are falling below 15 grams of fat, or exceeding 25 grams of fat, at meals, review the fat habit.

- If you notice processed foods are prominent in your meals, revisit the whole foods habit and try to replace some with unprocessed foods, which are often more satisfying for the calories and naturally facilitate overall reduction in energy intake.

- Liquid calories showing up? You know what to do, head back to the liquid calories chapter and commit to practicing that some more.

- Count up how many foods on your diary are treats, such as sweets, chocolate, ice cream, cookies, beer, wine, French fries or doughnuts. Even if you only have a very small portion ("just a taste"), you should be aware of it and consider it in your overall treat budget. If more than 10 percent of your calories are coming from treats, review your treats budget and focus on reducing intake of these foods to 10 percent or less of your overall calories.

- Compare weekends to weekdays. Are they consistent, or very different? Commonly, doing an honest three-day calorie count shows people that that they are eating appropriate amounts on weekdays and creating a suitable deficit, but eating considerably more calories on weekends and canceling out their deficit with caloric excess on Saturday and Sunday. If this is apparent in your log, commit to practicing your habits, including Hunger Mastery and Eating Just Enough as diligently on weekends as you do Monday through Friday.

Once you have picked one or more habits that you want to tune up, jot them down and start with one. Practice it for at least two weeks, working on it every day. If it takes longer than two weeks to master it and have it become automatic, take longer. Give yourself time; you are a work in progress. Work through each habit that you flagged from your food logging exercise, and you are likely to find that you are once again making progress.

Wendy's Story

Wendy's story is a great example of how to calorie count accurately, learn what you can and use it to inform your habit practice.

After a year of coaching, Wendy had lost more than 20 pounds but had hit a plateau when she began training for a half marathon. Despite an increased appetite, she felt like she was practicing all the habits consistently, aside from an occasional high-calorie meal on the weekend that didn't seem frequent enough to explain her weight's refusal to budge. Wendy was discouraged that maybe she just wouldn't be able to lose more weight. Feeling like she was doing everything right and seeing no progress on the scale was understandably upsetting after her patience and hard work. It just didn't seem fair. Wendy's fears are really common; many people have told me over the years that even though they know it's not supposed to work that way, they fear they will be the lone anomaly that cuts calories, gets into a substantial energy deficit and somehow can't lose weight.

I knew that was not the case, and I knew Wendy was more than capable of making changes. She had already made so many leaps and bounds, and it was clear she was a brave woman. We just needed to find out which habit (or habits) she thought she was doing right, but could do a little better. We decided that tracking calories would help settle the matter—we'd find out exactly how many calories she was eating and be able to see if she gained or lost weight. Since she is a math teacher, I knew Wendy would do a really good job of tracking her calories, and I was right.

She wanted to leave nothing to chance, her own bias or estimation. She measured everything, seldom ate out during the experiment, and when she did eat out, she only selected places with nutrition facts available.

With most calorie-logging software, a user can enter their initial body weight and choose a goal of maintaining weight (which gives the user a calorie target estimated to meet their energy needs) or losing weight (which cues the software to set the user's calorie goal lower than their estimated energy needs to encourage a daily energy deficit). Furthermore, the program Wendy used let her pick how much of a weight-loss goal rate she had, anywhere from a half pound a week to two pounds a week. Now, if she had asked me, I would have suggested Wendy aim for a half pound or one pound a week, which is typically concordant with the Hunger Mastery habit she had practiced of feeling hunger for 30 to 60 minutes before eating. But she didn't ask me, and Wendy's patience was running thin. With her half marathon approaching she wanted to move some extra pounds and she wanted to move them now. So she picked two pounds per week. She was not messing around.

When we talked on the phone to review the results of the experiment, Wendy had learned a ton. First and foremost, she had been able to do it! She had shown herself that she wasn't lacking self-control, that she could pick a hard task and see it all the way through. She also learned that it was hard to sort out what was a valid increase in hunger from her ramped up energy expenditure, and what was simply her mind thinking she should have more food or deserved more food because of all the running she did. Tracking also helped her silence the emotional part of her mind, which had frequently fought back against her healthy meal selections, saying, "That's not enough food! That's a starvation diet!" Armed with actual data, she could use the logical part of her mind to counteract with calm reason. "This is not a starvation amount of food, this is a 600-calorie meal which is absolutely enough for me and a suitable size." And it helped put her at ease and see what was an appropriate amount of food. Not being familiar with the calorie content of foods, she had her eyes opened to how concentrated some were in calories (Mexican food) while piles of veggies were quite the opposite. Wendy learned that while she had been including veggies with each meal, she hadn't been including large servings of them. While she was tracking her intake, she found that doubling the portion of fresh vegetables in her meals enabled her to get satisfied on fewer calories. Since she chose such an aggressive weight-loss goal, Wendy also got an abrupt lesson in how uncomfortable one needs to be to lose weight fast. Instead of feeling hunger for 30 to 60 minutes before each meal, she was tolerating hunger for two to three hours before each meal.

She chose such an extreme rate, she told me, because she wanted to know for darned sure if it was going to work or not. She suspected her body just wasn't able to lose fat for some reason, and she really wanted to prove her fears wrong. And she did! To both of our massive relief, Wendy lost two pounds the first week she was tracking. She felt it was worth it enough to do it for a second week, and lost another two pounds. She could finally see that she was not an anomaly, her body was just as willing to lose weight as everyone else's. Doing a detailed, accurate food log showed her what she needed to work on, and she got right to it: amping up the vegetables, choosing meals which were appropriately sized and quieting her emotional hungers in lieu of responding to only genuine physical hunger with food. She also was relieved to return to a moderate weight-loss pace and lose a half to one pound a week, feeling hunger for 30 to 60 minutes before each meal (which now seemed like a walk in the park).

Armed with bolstered confidence and several pounds lighter, Wendy tackled her first half marathon and, despite a sprained ankle, succeeded with a smile. The race proved again that while the going can be tough, nothing can stop her.

Lisa's Story

Lisa's story shows us some of the drawbacks of food logging and counting which make it a lousy long-term solution for weight management.

Like many of my clients, Lisa had a history of counting calories before we started working together. As she learned new nutrition habits, she was able to let go of counting and even stopped weighing herself. She felt good in her skin, comfortable with her food choices and confident that her habits were things she could do for the rest of her life. She moved on to living life instead of always trying to lose weight.

Then, something got in the way. Her pants got tight. And it wasn't just one pair, they all seemed to be getting snug. Even though Lisa was checking off each of her habits diligently every day, she seemed to be starting to gain weight back. And she was distraught over it. She urgently wanted to do something as soon as possible to make sure she could get those few pounds off because her clothes didn't fit and she didn't want to buy new ones. On one of our coaching calls we discussed the option of counting calories, and she was eager to return to it, feeling little faith in her ability to trust her appetite anymore. She commented to me that it was appealing because it offered a surefire way to maintain a deficit and get results. I hoped that tracking for a period of time would show her where in her habits her calories had increased above her needs, and that we could soon get her back to practicing her habits and not tracking.

Lisa did a thorough job of weighing and measuring everything she ate, and when we chatted about the experience, she had already drawn her own conclusions about the habits she needed to revisit. She realized that she hadn't been using Hunger Mastery and Eat Just Enough as well as she could be, and that all sorts of other factors were sneaking in and bumping up her food intake.

When she committed to feeling true physical hunger before each meal (which she had done successfully many times), she ate an amount of calories that was appropriate for gradual weight loss. However, occasionally she had fallen into the habit of eating because she felt she was "owed" more food, or because she had turned down something earlier in the day and thought she deserved to have some cookies after dinner. She also realized that her tendency to make the same meal over and over left her bored, and seeking more pleasure from food often meant tacking on sweets after her meals; even if she had physically had enough to eat, she felt shortchanged on enjoyment.

It also became apparent that calorie counting was making it harder to eat less! Having logging software tell her she was low on her calories for a day made it natural and easy to justify continuing to eat, even if she wasn't still hungry. She felt owed every calorie she had been allotted. Because entering ingredients from recipes was time consuming, her diet became even more repetitive as she repeated meals to save time on data entry. Packaged foods like protein bars were easier and more convenient to eat than weighing an apple or measuring out some yogurt. The repetitiveness and lack of enjoyment in her meals further made her crave hyper-palatable things like cookies and desserts for some fun and pleasure.

To help Lisa get back on track and have more success with Hunger Mastery and Eating Just Enough, we talked about the experience of hunger. Lisa felt that she was doing well with feeling hunger months ago, when she first practiced the Hunger Mastery habit, but lately she had been getting stressed and anxious when she felt it, and had not wanted to feel it for 30 minutes, so she often ate at the first sign of hunger. Further barring her progress, she often ate past fullness to prevent hunger from coming back soon, as it upset her so much. To help put hunger back in perspective as a normal, mild and easily managed sensation, I often compare the experience of hunger to how it feels to stay up an hour later than usual.

I asked Lisa if she ever stayed up past her usual bedtime and she said yes. "What does it feel like to get sleepy?" I asked. She responded, "It depends," and went on to explain that if it's a work night, getting sleepy makes her immediately anxious because she worries about how she'll function the next day, if she'll do poorly at her job, and she's likely to panic a little. But on a weekend, getting sleepy isn't a big deal at all and she'd be fine with feeling some heavy eyelids or yawning, since she can sleep in the next day. "That is exactly what happens with hunger," I explained. When we interpret hunger (or sleepiness) as something that will cause a problem, as a dangerous or "bad" feeling, it triggers anxiety and stress, which are far more unpleasant than the actual hunger itself. Mild sensations of hollowness in your stomach aren't hard to bear, but anxiety, worry and doomsday predictions that we can attach to hunger are. When we let go of associations and just experience hunger like any other feeling, we realize we can handle it without a problem and don't need to run from it or fear it.

Lisa seemed really heartened to get back to practicing Hunger Mastery with this new mind-set, and within a day, sent me a happy e-mail that she was doing better than ever at feeling hunger without judging it, and being able to leave a few bites at each meal. Seeing that her repetitive meals were leaving her shortchanged on enjoyment, she committed to including a wider variety of food in her meals and looking for joy and fulfillment in other areas of her life, not just at the table.

Furthermore, the experiment reminded Lisa how stressful it is to track calories. It was like a glimpse into an unhappy former life. While it was challenging to use her hunger and satiety cues to guide her eating when she wasn't tracking calories, once she was plugging everything into a program and having numbers flashed in her face, it became impossible. She remembered how, when she tracked calories for months on end, she had zero sense of ever feeling hungry or full; all she felt was "constant low-level anxiety after eating that I have to get to my computer or phone and log items immediately or risk forgetting what I ate. It became a compulsion and I constantly checked my tally to plan what I could eat next, regardless of my true hunger signals." She also noticed that she fixated on particular food items, stocking up on the lowest-calorie foods and obsessing about junk food, ate more processed foods because they were easy to track and avoided cooking recipes with many (healthy) ingredients such as a fancy colorful salad or multi-vegetable soup.

These experiences aren't unique to Lisa; I've heard hundreds of people recount similar experiences. Eating the same thing all the time feels monotonous, depriving, and easily triggers a desire to binge or overeat. For this reason I cannot stress enough that a calorie counting exercise should be performed only for a short length of time to increase awareness. As soon as you can, return to practicing habits.

Tracy's Story

What we can all learn from Tracy is that calorie counting is potentially a psychologically dangerous thing. Especially if you had negative experiences in the past from dieting, weighing and measuring out foods or having a list in front of you of what you're going to eat today can make even the sanest, level-headed eater get twitchy. If you think of it as a diet, it is a diet, even if you set it up yourself.

Tracy started working with me after being on an extreme diet program recommended by her doctor. The diet was a ketogenic, very-low-carbohydrate program, which also included fasting most of the day and eating only one meal. Her doctor had urged Tracy to follow this extreme diet to help keep her blood sugar down, but after months of not being able to eat even a piece of fruit or a tomato (because fruit and most vegetables were not allowed) Tracy's quality of life was suffering. When the restriction became too much, she would binge on desserts, cookies, candy and cereal, all the things her doctor had forbidden her to eat. And afterward, she would feel remorseful and worried about what these onslaughts of sugar did to her body. She visualized all the sugar and carbohydrates poisoning her, hurting her kidneys and blood vessels, making her fatter and pushing her closer to diabetes. So she would go back to the strict diet again, allowing only meat and green vegetables, and only one meal per day. And she could keep that up for days or weeks at a time, but inevitably, the unfairness of not being allowed to eat "normally" would get under her skin again, and the cycle would repeat.

As Tracy and I talked about normalizing her eating, we discussed learning to rely on appetite and satiety cues to eat three meals a day, and venture into the forbidden food groups: fruits, colorful vegetables, whole grains and dairy foods were back on the menu! Tracy was eager but also scared that she would go overboard and eat massive quantities of food, since the variety she could enjoy now was simply staggering. She had some anxiety over eating with the lack of structure and asked if she could count calories just to keep an eye on things and make sure she wasn't eating 5,000 calories a day.

While I typically dissuade clients from counting calories, I thought in this case, if it provided Tracy some reassurance, it might be helpful. I hoped that 1) it would help her feel more comfortable that she could eat any food, even sweets, and still have a level of carbohydrates which was healthy and balanced at the end of the day, and 2) that she'd see her calorie total would be reasonable if she remembered to eat only when hungry and stop at satisfied.

The first day of calorie counting was an utter disaster. Tracy planned out her meals the night before using a calorie counting website, and being a detail-oriented person, selected exactly how many grams of each food she would eat the following day. Breakfast went okay … but shortly after, things went downhill. Trying to stick to her own plan felt like being back on a restrictive diet. She felt stressed and rebellious. What if she didn't want the salad and half sandwich she had allotted herself for lunch? Why couldn't she have something else? She ended up throwing out her plan, going out to eat with her friends, overeating and not feeling good about the choices she made at all. She felt out of control and reactive, not at all the calm, happy eater she wanted to be. We abandoned calorie counting then and there in favor of a flexible meal template based on her habits.

Lessons to take home from Tracy's experience: remember to be flexible, and don't make rigid future plans to eat specific foods and hit exact calorie or macronutrient amounts. If you lock yourself into the "plan," it feels like you can't go out for lunch if your boss invites you. If the leftover salmon you are supposed to eat for dinner tonight doesn't seem too appealing when you get home, you're stuck. And that's likely to put you into a bad mood. To preserve your sanity if you do decide to count calories for a period of time, use it as a backup check, and just eat as you normally do. Rather than focus on the numbers, keep your eye on the big picture: practicing your habits.

TROUBLESHOOT 6: I'M FULL OF EXCUSES!

Just as negative thoughts and feelings can undermine your motivation, excuses and rationalizations can also lure you from your intended behaviors when temptation arises. I'm going to introduce you to a dozen different types of sabotaging thoughts you might encounter, and for each one, how to fight back. The more you believe sabotaging self-talk and act accordingly (allowing yourself to make the excuse and deviate from your intention), the more pervasive the problem becomes. However, once you can hear them loud and clear and know immediately what they are, you have the upper hand to refute them and not take the bait.

Note: please understand that this section is in no way meant to be taken in a drill sergeant's "No excuses!" tone. Sometimes there is an excuse. If I were at a loved one's bedside in the emergency room, I would not consider nutrition habits my top priority. "I want to be here at my mother's bedside, I don't care if I get dinner or what it is" is not a sabotaging thought. That's just having priorities! There is a time and place to put other things first. The types of excuses I'll talk about here are ones that rank rather low on validity and truth, and thus are good ones to question.

DENYING THE DAMAGE

This type of sabotaging thought denies that a poor food choice counts, or makes us think it's "not so bad." It functions to prevent us from feeling our cognitive dissonance (the fact that what we're about to do is at odds with our goal). It also gives us permission to go for immediate gratification.

Examples

- It's only a bite/sliver … there are only three bites left.
- I biked hard, I earned the extra calories.
- It's not mine so it doesn't count.
- A few bites won't hurt.
- No one saw me eat it, therefore it doesn't count.
- It wasn't on my plate, therefore it doesn't count.
- It won't make a difference.
- This is the last time I will eat this.
- I'm not overweight, so I can totally have this treat, no big deal.

- I'm usually really good, so this little treat won't make a big difference.
- It's just one meal.
- It's just one bite.
- Today's a write-off so let's have at 'er.
- There's barely any left; I'll just finish it.
- I already messed up at lunch, so just blow dinner too!
- I'm just going to finish this off so it won't be around to tempt me ....
- Oh, I'm building muscles; I don't have to watch what I eat.
- This little piece of this or that won't really do any damage.
- Just this once I'll make an exception.
- I'll just have one. That's not very many calories, so I can afford it.
- I'll skip dinner later.
- I'll make it up tomorrow.
- I have lost some weight this week, so even though eating this will set me back a bit the overall trend is still good.
- I can get away with it.
- I worked out hard today, so I can eat this/that/the other.
- It won't count if I don't count it.

How to Fight Back

Use the truth, because every one of these is a lie! All food counts. You are always in control and responsible for what goes in your mouth, no matter what you ate earlier, if it's your birthday or if you call it a cheat day. (Your fat cells don't know it's a cheat day, and they definitely still work on holidays.) You are never "so off track" that the only thing left to do is keep eating junk—you always have the steering wheel in your hands. If you tend to promise yourself you'll make it up tomorrow, skip dinner or start Monday, ask yourself how much evidence you have that this is true. Has that worked before, when you have made that same bargain? Have you ever actually eaten just one bite?

Furthermore, self-imposed scarcity (aka dieting) is never helpful. Swearing you will start a diet tomorrow will only increase your fears of impending restriction and make you continue eating. Better to stop, take a deep breath and remind yourself that this food will not be gone from the face of the earth, ever. You could always have more tomorrow. In fact, you can't eat all of the ice cream on the planet tonight, so don't bother trying, please. If you are going to get control over your eating, it's not going to be because you exhausted the world's supply of Chunky Monkey; it's going to be because you learned to not be controlled by sabotaging thoughts.

NUTRITIONAL REASONING/HUNGER PREVENTION

Rather than denying that a particular food decision is damaging, these types of sabotaging thoughts go further to invent an upside to eating the food, such as a nutritional benefit. They function similarly to "Denying the Damage" thoughts, in that they give us reason to not feel so bad about eating the food. Additionally, this type of sabotaging thought often strikes people who have a fear of being hungry, preventing them from getting the calorie deficit needed to lose weight.

Examples
- It's good for me, so I should eat it.
- It's a healthy alternative food. Almond butter, almond meal, coconut anything.
- It's sugar-free.
- It's low-fat.
- It's a cheat day.
- I might get low blood sugar during my workout later.
- Post-workout carbs are good for recovery.
- I wonder when I will be able to eat again because I'm super busy.
- I will eat this because it will keep me full for a while.
- There might not be anything available where I'm going later.
- If I don't eat enough, my body will go into starvation mode and I won't lose weight.
- This will balance out my macros.

How to Fight Back

More facts! Calories count; it doesn't matter if a food is low in fat or sugar-free or Paleo or gluten-free, they *all* can make you gain weight. Eating more of a specific food or nutrient does not "undo" or balance out other things that you ate. You do need more fuel and carbohydrates if you are physically active, but you don't need to push past satiety or include high-sugar processed foods. Last, starvation mode does not exist. There is no point at which eating fewer calories will halt weight loss. If you aren't hungry, don't let this myth trick you into eating (because that really *will* get in the way of your weight loss).

REWARD/ENTITLEMENT

This type of sabotaging thought may be a signal that somewhere else in your life, you might be shortchanging yourself. I'm not going to say that's always the case, but it's pretty common to use food rewards in place of other, more gratifying ones. For example, if you really want to buy a particular item, but feel like it's too much money, you might buy food as a cheap alternative. Food thrills are accessible and inexpensive.

Often it's not a physical object you desire, but a feeling or experience such as being good to yourself, being indulgent, being irresponsible or having what you want for once. In working with my one-on-one coaching clients, we often discover that previously uncontrollable desires for specific foods lessen greatly when we work on reducing other self-sacrificial behaviors. As one put it marvelously, "I have never been rebellious, other than with food. I do what everyone says and wants, always go with the flow. Always the good girl. I never would have thought in a million years that learning to speak my mind and stand up for what I want could lessen my desires for junk food and help me lose fat, but it *did*."

Examples
- This food is my reward for reaching a goal.
- I deserve it.
- I had a bad/stressful/boring day, I deserve to eat this.

- I worked hard, so I deserve a treat.
- I've been good all week.
- I had an awesome workout and have earned a reward.

How to Fight Back

When you notice your thoughts turning to "deserving" or "earning" food, remind yourself that all foods are ethically neutral. It's just food. You wouldn't think you "deserve to wear yellow today," would you? So why would you deserve less healthy food after a particularly hard day at the office? I'd replace it with "I deserve to feel good about what I eat tonight," "I deserve to be good to myself when it seems like other people are all giving me a hard time" or simply, "I deserve results, health, confidence and self-trust." Really, compared to the junk food your sabotaging thoughts are trying to justify, aren't you actually worthy of something far better?

I suggest not using food as a reward as much as you can possibly avoid it, for yourself or your children. If you choose to eat a cookie, say, "I'm choosing to eat a cookie," or "I'm going to eat a cookie," not, "I'm going to reward myself with a cookie" or "I've earned a cookie." You eat something or don't, leave the ethical words out.

A feeling of "entitlement to eat crap" is often the aftereffect of feeling like you were unfairly treated or infringed upon previously. Try looking backward in the chain of events of that day or week, to see if there are any circumstances in which you cut yourself short or lacked assertiveness, or could have treated yourself with more respect.

THE ILLUSION OF CONFLICTING VALUES (SUCH AS FAIRNESS AND FRUGALITY)

We all want to live in line with our values. When we don't, we lose a bit of integrity and self-esteem. It's normal and healthy to have values that matter to you other than nutrition, and this type of sabotaging thought plays on those. Many people value saving money or not wasting food, values that can appear to be in conflict with the immediate behavior that would be best for weight loss. Fairness, in particular, is an ideal which many people regard. If we feel like everything "should be" fair and equitable (and therefore we should all be able to eat as much as everyone else), that can also lead to food decisions that thwart our weight loss efforts.

Examples
- Everyone else eats it and isn't fat.
- Everyone else is eating/drinking that.
- Other people don't have to miss out, why should I?
- So and so can eat it.
- If I don't finish it I'm wasting food.
- I need to clear my plate or I am wasting money and food.
- It's a good deal to buy a large pizza, so we can use the leftovers.
- They don't let us take home leftovers here.
- We paid for all three courses.

How to Fight Back

Be careful of false logic. You don't actually *save* any money by eating extra at a buffet, and you don't lose any money by tossing out the last few bites of popcorn in the bowl. The starving children in Africa don't get any more food by you eating everything on your plate and gaining weight. It may seem unfair that Sally can eat a lot more than you and not gain weight, but your overeating doesn't restore the metabolic fairness of the universe. It makes your pants tighter.

CAVING TO OTHERS' JUDGMENT OR OPINION

We like to think of ourselves as nice people. This type of sabotaging thought is rooted, just like the previous one, in our values. When we act with other people's feelings in mind, it preserves our notions of ourselves as kind and considerate people. Unfortunately, it can be an easy scapegoat, giving us our own permission to eat unhealthy foods. Or, it can cause the stressful feeling that you have to eat something you truly don't want to.

Examples

- My mom/sister/friend made it for me, therefore I must eat it to acknowledge their care.
- Gotta eat it because if I don't, my parents will think I don't love them.
- I want to help the Girl Scouts (evil little girls that they are).
- This lovely person took the time to make this—one of my favorites—just for me. I can't not eat any.
- I don't want to stick out from the crowd.
- If I don't eat what everyone else is eating, they'll think I'm weird.
- My kids made these and will be so disappointed if I don't have one.

How to Fight Back

When it comes to loved ones, I remind my clients, "People don't care how much you eat, they care how much you care." While you may feel like there is a lot of attention on you and your plate, seldom do people actually notice if you don't eat what they brought. Do you remember what any of your relatives ate at Thanksgiving last year? If you really do want to enjoy something your kids or coworker gave you as a present, you can enjoy it with your next meal, you don't have to consume it immediately. What will make the gift giver happiest is a heartfelt, genuine thanks, not seeing you scarf it down on the spot.

CHOICE BLINDNESS

An interesting thing I've learned about the human mind is how we love to feel in control (so we have power), yet we equally adore feeling like we have no control (so we don't risk blame). Denying or disowning the control we have is appealing at times because it relieves us of responsibility. All of the sabotaging thoughts in this category are actually false, because they are based on the idea that we had no choice but to eat unhealthy things. Really, what these are saying is, "It's not my fault!" so we can slough our guilt. The truth is that we choose to eat whatever we do. Own it.

Examples

- I forgot to prep my food, so I need to fall back on my old strategies.
- I don't have time.
- I need it.
- I'm too tired to cook.
- I'll go CRAZY if I don't eat it NOW!
- I tried everything I could to distract myself but it didn't work. At least I tried.
- These thoughts won't leave me alone … I can't help it. I HAVE to.
- I can't say no.
- I'm powerless around chocolate. I'm addicted.

How to Fight Back

Repeat after me: I am always in control. No food is forced into my mouth against my will. I can always take steps to find a better option or decide not to eat. I am as responsible for what goes in my mouth as I am for what comes out of it. I may decide to not go to undue efforts to obtain healthier food (for example, at a catered event where leaving isn't socially acceptable), but I am always in control of how much I eat, even in rare circumstances when I don't have control over what's available. For those times, I can usually plan ahead and exert more of my personal responsibility over my food choices. I will not go crazy, lose my mind or otherwise self-destruct without a certain food. Telling myself "I can't resist (trigger food)" is just giving up, and denies me the chance to strengthen my self-control and work on my relationship with that food. Instead, I can acknowledge that that food has been a problem for me in the past, but doesn't always have to be.

Do long days happen, when you might feel too tired to cook? Sure. They happen to me too! You can choose to eat out, you can choose something healthy from a delivery menu or sit-down restaurant, you can choose to cook anyway, you can choose to plan ahead and have the fridge/freezer stocked with ready-to-heat meals, or you can choose to order delivery pizza and fried wings. Choose it and own it.

CONTEXT ASSOCIATIONS

Associations are links in our mind between two unrelated things. This type of thought sabotage happens when we associate food, or a specific type of food, with a particular context. That context might be an event, holiday, time or place. It might also be the company of a specific person.

Examples
- I'm on vacation.
- It's the weekend.
- It's a snow day.
- It's new.
- It's my birthday.
- It's a holiday.

How to Fight Back

Recognize that situation, time and place don't actually change the impact of food on your body. Everything you eat counts the same, so make decisions with your usual values in mind, as you do in other settings.

GIVING FOOD POSITIVE SUPERPOWERS

These are also a type of association, but unlike contextual associations, we associate food with a special power or trait, which it doesn't have. These special powers can be positive or negative. Negative superpowers can make us believe that eating particular foods makes us ethically bad in some way, which can lead to food phobias or a limited list of "safe" foods. Attributing positive special powers to food is more commonly associated with weight-loss trouble. To see the positive association in one's own sabotaging thought, you often have to read between the lines a bit. In the examples below you can pick out associations linking food with love, trust, fun, comfort, energy, calm and peace.

Examples

- Food is the only thing that I can use to prove that I am loved/loveable. I am the only one who knows/loves me enough to provide exactly the food I crave in this moment.
- Food is the only thing that has ever been faithful to me.
- It will make me feel better.
- I'm antsy, eating will help.
- I had a really rotten day and need some consolation.
- It will satisfy me.
- I need to have some fun on this weekend away.
- I want comfort food./This is my comfort food.
- Chocolate has always been my best antidepressant/antianxiety/anti-exhaustion medicine.
- I need the energy: a sugar boost, a caffeine boost, or both, in the case of chocolate.
- I'm so tired and I have no energy. If I eat something (especially chocolate), maybe it will give me some energy and make me feel better.
- I'm going through a rough patch, and I am being kind to myself by eating _____.
- I will be miserable without it.
- If I resist it I'll be sad and unsatisfied.

How to Fight Back

Remember that food is just food. It's not a surrogate, replacement or requisite for love, joy, adventure or anything else you desire in life. Eating has a very limited capacity to change your emotional state, so an expectation that eating will drastically improve a bad day is often a setup for disappointment. Food is great at fixing hunger, but that's about it. Think of other things that bring you comfort and relaxation, like connecting with someone you love, taking some quiet time or petting your dog or cat. Furthermore, you are highly unlikely to be miserable without a food if you choose to pass on it. Have you ever *actually* found yourself profoundly regretful of something you didn't eat? Have you ever heard someone say, "There was apple pie and ice cream, but I decided to have tea instead. Man, I am so disappointed! Why did I do that?!"

IDENTITY ISSUES

Foods and eating behaviors can be a way we communicate our identity. We may also identify ourselves by the foods we don't eat. Our food choices can be worsened by sabotaging thoughts which confirm our current identity ("I'm a chocoholic"), make us feel closer to an identity we want ("I want to be the fun mom") or make us feel more separation from an identity we don't want ("I don't want to be one of those uptight dieters"). In those who have battled eating disorders previously, eating unhealthy foods can be a way to distance oneself from the old disordered identity.

Examples
- I should be happy with what I look like and not try to change. I should be a confident woman.
- I hate low-carb people anyway.
- I'm a happy eater. There are no rules or restrictions.
- I'm (insert ethnicity here), we eat a lot of (insert food here).
- I'm not on a diet.
- I want to be the "fun mom" just this once.
- I'm someone who can't stick to a diet.
- I am leaving my disordered past behind, pass the cake around again!
- I have the freedom to eat what I want and I am eating this to prove it.

How to Fight Back

Your identity is who you are, not defined by what's on your plate. Eating white rice doesn't make you "more Chinese." Food choices make poor vehicles through which to deliver a political opinion or message. Whether you are trying to say that you are not on a diet or that you disagree with the treatment of women in your office culture, people rarely interpret our lunchbox contents as such. Better to make your impact on the world with other actions, and prove things to yourself by the character qualities you display, not the dessert you order.

ABANDONMENT OF THE GOAL

To work toward a goal, we need two fundamental beliefs: *It is worth it* and *I can do it*. When we start to lose faith in one or both of those necessary elements, we might abandon the goal. In some form or another, this type of thought implies it's either not worth it to lose weight or that we cannot do it. It may also take the form of not really needing to lose weight. Quick on the tails of this thought, the rhetorical question, "So why bother?" often follows.

Examples
- I'm naturally overweight. There's nothing I can do about it.
- I have a slow metabolism.
- I suck at nutrition anyway.
- Tomorrow I can start again anyway.
- What difference does it make? I will fail eventually.
- I'll never have the body I want, so why bother?
- Everyone tells me I look good already.
- My husband (friends, kids, dog) love me as I am.
- It's too hard.
- I'm tired of saying no.
- No one really cares about my weight, so why should I?
- My body stays the same anyway.

How to Fight Back

It can be helpful to remind yourself of any evidence that you do, in fact, care about losing weight. When faced with "I don't care about my weight right now" thinking, you may correct yourself, "I might not care right *now*, but tomorrow morning or Saturday when I weigh in I sure will care." "I cared enough to hire a coach, to join a gym, to pay a trainer, so I think 99 percent of the time I do care; let me not get sidetracked by this one second in time when I might not feel that caring." You may also remind yourself of the reasons you wanted to lose weight or eat better by having them written down—seeing them in black and white can help you remember *why* it's worth it to you to make a positive change.

If you are starting to feel like it's too much effort to stick to your plan (and therefore not worth it), take a critical look at how many hours or minutes of the day you are truly having to try very hard. If you are thinking "I am tired of this 24/7 job!" you might feel a bit different when you calm down and see it's really only hard for a couple hours in the afternoon and maybe the 30 minutes after you get home from work. So for a small percentage of your day you are exerting some effort. Much of the day you are fine. Maybe right now, when the "This is too hard" thoughts are popping up, is just one of those isolated hard moments.

As for sabotaging thoughts that center on not being able to succeed, I would turn that right around as, "Thoughts like that that lead me to eat junk are *exactly* why I haven't been able to succeed." I'll also point out that after working with hundreds of people, I can verify that no one reaches a state of carrying excess weight by destiny alone. Sure, genetics and parenting influence make it harder for some than others, but it's never true that there is nothing you can do about it. If you have excess weight to lose, there is something you can do about it. It starts with not believing those false thoughts that you have a broken metabolism or that even eating healthier would somehow keep you from losing fat.

LIMITED OPPORTUNITY/SCARCITY

That which is rare is perceived as more valuable. Reminding ourselves, or fibbing to ourselves, that we'll never have this again or not for a really, really long time, can help tip the scale of "eat it or don't eat it" in favor of eating it. Several sabotaging thought examples below also hint that eating a certain food now represents sticking up for ourselves.

Examples
- It's here and available and I might not get to eat it later.
- I'll never be at this restaurant again.

- If I don't get to these muffins, someone else will take them! So I have to eat them now before anyone else eats my treats.
- Now's my chance.

How to Fight Back

Chances to eat indulgent, delicious foods abound. While you may not be at this same restaurant again or anytime soon, there will be plenty of other opportunities to eat both healthy and not-so-healthy foods. So what if you miss an opportunity to eat something? Is missing the last store-bought muffin from the break room really a tragedy? Imagine yourself 10 or 20 years from now, looking back. Can you see yourself saying, "I wish I had eaten that ice cream sandwich when I had the chance; life would have been different" ... or is it more likely you would have regretted not living healthfully? When you say no to one thing, you also say yes to something. By choosing to not miss out on food you think is "special," you might be missing out on having weight-loss success. Note: it's not that you need to turn down all treats to lose weight. But you can't take every opportunity to eat them.

QUANTITY SABOTEURS

Once you're in the midst of eating something you know is a bad food decision, the game isn't even over. With a healthy, logical (if somewhat utopian) inner dialogue, we'd realize, "Wait, I don't want to be eating this ice cream! It's more important to me to feel good about my body and meet my weight-loss goal!" And we'd stop. I've saved this class of sabotaging thought for last because it's a bit different from the others, which typically get us into trouble. The quantity saboteurs actually keep us going once we're in trouble. These are the bad boys that twist our thinking so much that we decide we'll just continue the self-harming behavior.

Examples
- This food is so tempting ... I need to eat it up so it won't tempt me anymore.
- I better eat a lot because I will probably not let myself have it again.

- This is my last chance to eat everything off-limits.
- I'd better eat all of this and get rid of it.
- There's only a little of this left, so I might as well finish it off.
- There's so much of this, no one will notice if I have a little more.

How to Fight Back

Remind yourself that if you want to get rid of the remainder of a food, you can toss it in the trash or down the sink; you don't have to eat it. This isn't ever your last chance to have a food because you aren't going on a diet tomorrow. You aren't doing that anymore. Considering whether someone else will or won't notice what you ate is unimportant. *You* know. What is important is how you feel about your eating choices. Even if no one else notices what you ate, if it makes you feel crummy or anything less than proud, that's a bigger thing to tune in to. And no food mistake gets better by continuing to eat, so if you've already started down a path you don't like, just put the brakes on, remind yourself it's no big deal, forgive yourself and move on. If you know there's no massive guilt trip coming, there's less incentive to keep eating to delay it.

OTHER TIPS FOR OPTIMAL RESULTS

Log your habit practice every single day. Having utilized this system with hundreds of people, I can confirm that those who diligently log their habit practice every day achieve far greater results than the people who only record sporadically. Your log will not be as accurate as it can be if you only open it once every few days and try to remember what you did in the past. Even if you could remember with 100 percent accuracy, you'd be missing out on an important part of the process: reading your desired behavior list each day, to refresh your commitment and remind yourself what you are working on. If losing fat is important to you, remind yourself that you can take a couple minutes to read your checklist every day to increase your chances of succeeding. If you forget your notebook, use another method of recording (such as your phone or e-mail), or set reminders in your calendar. You can use a spreadsheet such as Google docs and set it as your Internet browser home page, or purchase a habit tracking app such as Habit List.

Expect imperfection while doing your best. You don't need 100 percent perfection with these habits to lose weight, so don't panic if you miss a habit checkmark every once in a while. Think about practicing them as much of the time as possible, and remember that like anything else you practice, it's going to get easier with more repetition.

Consider teaming up. If you have a friend or family member working on the Lean Habits with you, you can share the experience and support each other. Stop by the Lean Habits Facebook group to meet other people using the system and share your insights.

RELAPSE PREVENTION

As you've started to use the Lean Habits you've read about in this book, you've probably made some considerable changes. Some of those habits you are changing may be things you did for decades, but here you are, settling into new ones that should be getting more automatic with each passing day. It's pretty amazing, actually, to think that a lifetime of overeating, eating emotionally or eating without thinking doesn't destine us to continue the same behaviors forever. How incredible that we can always, always change our course.

The human brain exhibits remarkable neuroplasticity, the ability to reorganize itself throughout a lifetime by changing neural pathways. This capacity, however, also means that your new healthy habits aren't carved in stone. To avoid backsliding or slipping into new unhealthy patterns, I'll discuss in this section how to preserve your new habits so they stay with you, grow with you and help you not only achieve but keep your leanness for life.

PREVENTION FIRST

Weight regain, like a house fire, is best prevented. You wouldn't leave candles burning when you went out to dinner or pile newspapers on the radiator, and you probably have a smoke detector or two installed. You've planned ahead so that just in case a fire did start, you could stop it as early as possible, minimize the damage and prevent the whole house from burning down.

Likewise, you don't have to regain 10 pounds before realizing, "I think I might be straying from my prior habit consistency." Noticing the early signs of habit drift allow you to adjust before you've backtracked significantly.

When I graduate clients from my coaching program, the last coaching phone call is focused on the art of maintenance. Maintaining the very same habits that got a person to their goal weight is essential for keeping them at that weight. We make a plan ahead of time for what they'll look out for as indicators, red flags of things changing in an unfavorable direction. And for each indicator, we make a plan for what action they'll take if they notice it. I'm going to do that same exercise with you now, so you are prepared and don't have to make a plan in haste and panic *after* things are already going south.

NAME YOUR INDICATORS

We organize indicators into four categories: Behaviors, Thoughts, Feelings and Physical Cues. For each of these, think about and write down one or more indicators that would tell *you* that you may be sliding a bit further from your healthy lifestyle than you'd like.

Behaviors: If you had a surveillance camera and could watch yourself on videotape, what behaviors would signal to you that you aren't acting in a way that helps you maintain your results? Would you be staring into the fridge late at night? Would you be wandering the junk food aisles of the grocery store, buying things and saying, "It's just for the kids"? Would you be exercising for the second time in a day out of punishment?

Thoughts: Write down the thoughts you might catch in your internal dialogue that would be warning signs to you. Examples might be: "I blew it already, I'll start again Monday," or "Oh, this 1,500-calorie meal plan in this magazine looks like it's worth a try."

Feelings: Experiencing certain emotions around food, eating or exercising can signify that something isn't right. Indicators that our clients commonly list in this category are shame and secrecy around eating treats, panic or anxiety regarding hunger, regret after eating or disappointment with themselves.

Physical Cues: Your body itself will help provide information on how your habits are. Weight gain is one of the most popular indicators, and many clients choose to keep themselves accountable by committing to monitoring their weight at regular intervals. Other indicators that you can be aware of include digestion, energy levels, physical performance in the gym, sleep quality and how your clothes fit.

Take a few minutes to write down one or more indicators in each of these categories that signify to you that it's time to take action to get back on track.

PLAN ACTIONS FOR EACH INDICATOR

There's more than one way to get back on track. For each indicator, plan what you will do immediately when you notice it. Here are some examples:

Behavioral Indicator: Hanging by the buffet and eating too much at a party.
Action: As soon as I realize it, walk away. Get a glass of water and sit down away from the food.

Thought Indicator: "I might as well have dessert, I already ate too much."
Action: Stop that thought in its tracks, order a coffee or tea and remind myself that adding more calories to a dietary mistake doesn't help and makes things worse.

Feeling Indicator: Fear of attending a wedding because I don't trust myself to not overeat.
Action: Touch base with a supportive friend or e-mail my coach. Remind myself of my successes and ask my date to help be supportive.

Physical Cues Indicator: "Ooof, my pants are tight."
Action: Use my habit tracker for a week to see if I am eating between meals, not being hungry for 30 to 60 minutes before each time I eat or including too many treats.

It's in your hands now, you've got a road map to follow and a proven path that others have traveled before you. There is no need to rush, so enjoy the Lean Habits journey and at every step of the way, be patient, be kind to yourself, and be open-minded. Don't be afraid to circle back to previous chapters and re-read portions of this book as you focus on one habit at a time. If you have questions or need help, ask for it. Changing all 16 habits at once is possible, but I know you can do this, one habit at a time.

RESOURCES

Agus, M. S., Swain, J. F., Larson, C. L., Eckert, E. A., & Ludwig, D. S. (2000). Dietary composition and physiologic adaptations to energy restriction. *American Journal of Clinical Nutrition*, 71(4), 901–7. Retrieved from http://ajcn.nutrition.org/content/71/4/901.full

Allirot, X., Seyssel, K., Saulais, L., Roth, H., Charrié, A., Drai, J., . . . Laville, M. (2014). Effects of a breakfast spread out over time on the food intake at lunch and the hormonal responses in obese men. *Physiology & Behavior*, 127, 37–44. doi:10.1016/j.physbeh.2014.01.004

Aragon, A. A., & Schoenfeld, B. J. (2013). Nutrient timing revisited: Is there a post-exercise anabolic window? *Journal of the International Society of Sports Nutrition*, 10(1), 5. doi:10.1186/1550-2783-10-5

Armstrong, L. E. (2012). Challenges of linking chronic dehydration and fluid consumption to health outcomes. *Nutrition Reviews*, 70 Suppl 2, S121–27. doi:10.1111/j.1753-4887.2012.00539.x

Avena, N. M., Murray, S., & Gold, M. S. (2013). Comparing the effects of food restriction and overeating on brain reward systems. *Experimental Gerontology*, 48(10), 1062–67. doi:10.1016/j.exger.2013.03.006

Beglinger, C., & Degen, L. (2004). Fat in the intestine as a regulator of appetite—role of CCK. *Physiology & Behavior*, 83(4), 617–21. doi:10.1016/j.physbeh.2004.07.031

Belza, A., Ritz, C., Sørensen, M. Q., Holst, J. J., Rehfeld, J. F., & Astrup, A. (2013). Contribution of gastroenteropancreatic appetite hormones to protein-induced satiety. *American Journal of Clinical Nutrition*, 97(5), 980–89. doi:10.3945/ajcn.112.047563

Bertéus Forslund, H., Torgerson, J. S., Sjöström, L., & Lindroos, A.K. (2005). Snacking frequency in relation to energy intake and food choices in obese men and women compared to a reference population. *International Journal of Obesity (2005)*, 29(6), 711–19. doi:10.1038/sj.ijo.0802950

Blechert, J., Goltsche, J. E., Herbert, B. M., & Wilhelm, F. H. (2013). Eat your troubles away: Electrocortical and experiential correlates of food image processing are related to emotional eating style and emotional state. *Biological Psychology*, 96C, 94–101. doi:10.1016/j.biopsycho.2013.12.007

Blundell, J. E., & King, N. A. (1996). Overconsumption as a cause of weight gain: Behavioural-physiological interactions in the control of food intake (appetite). *Ciba Foundation Symposium*, 201, 138–54; discussion 154–58, 188–93. Retrieved from http://www.ncbi.nlm.nih.gov/pubmed/9017279

Bohon, C., Stice, E., & Spoor, S. (2009). Female emotional eaters show abnormalities in consummatory and anticipatory food reward: A functional magnetic resonance imaging study. *The International Journal of Eating Disorders*, 42(3), 210–21. doi:10.1002/eat.20615

Boschmann, M., Steiniger, J., Hille, U., Tank, J., Adams, F., Sharma, A. M., . . . Jordan, J. (2003). Water-induced thermogenesis. *Journal of Clinical Endocrinology and Metabolism*, 88(12), 6015–19. doi:10.1210/jc.2003-030780

Bowen, J., Noakes, M., & Clifton, P. M. (2006). Appetite regulatory hormone responses to various dietary proteins differ by body mass index status despite similar reductions in ad libitum energy intake. *Journal of Clinical Endocrinology and Metabolism*, 91(8), 2913–19. doi:10.1210/jc.2006-0609

Brown, C. M., Dulloo, A. G., & Montani, J.-P. (2006). Water-induced thermogenesis reconsidered: The effects of osmolality and water temperature on energy expenditure after drinking. *The Journal of Clinical Endocrinology and Metabolism*, 91(9), 3598–602. doi:10.1210/jc.2006-0407

Burdakov, D., Luckman, S. M., & Verkhratsky, A. (2005). Glucose-sensing neurons of the hypothalamus. *Philosophical Transactions of the Royal Society of London. Series B, Biological Sciences*, 360(1464), 2227–35. doi:10.1098/rstb.2005.1763

Buxton, O. M., Pavlova, M., Reid, E. W., Wang, W., Simonson, D. C., & Adler, G. K. (2010). Sleep restriction for 1 week reduces insulin sensitivity in healthy men. *Diabetes*, 59(9), 2126–33. doi:10.2337/db09-0699

Cameron, J. D., Cyr, M.-J., & Doucet, E. (2010). Increased meal frequency does not promote greater weight loss in subjects who were prescribed an 8-week equi-energetic energy-restricted diet. *British Journal of Nutrition*, 103(8), 1098–101. doi:10.1017/S0007114509992984

Chao, Y.-H., Yang, C.-C., & Chiou, W.-B. (2012). Food as ego-protective remedy for people experiencing shame: Experimental evidence for a new perspective on weight-related shame. *Appetite*, 59(2), 570–75. doi:10.1016/j.appet.2012.07.007

Chapelot, D. (2011). The role of snacking in energy balance : A biobehavioral approach. *Journal of Nutrition*, (7). doi:10.3945/jn.109.114330.158

Chen, L., Appel, L. J., Loria, C., Lin, P.-H., Champagne, C. M., Elmer, P. J., . . . Caballero, B. (2009). Reduction in consumption of sugar-sweetened beverages is associated with weight loss: The PREMIER trial. *The American Journal of Clinical Nutrition*, 89(5), 1299–306. doi:10.3945/ajcn.2008.27240

Chin-Chance, C., Polonsky, K. S., & Schoeller, D. A. (2000). Twenty-four-hour leptin levels respond to cumulative short-term energy imbalance and predict subsequent intake. *Journal of Clinical Endocrinology and Metabolism*, 85(8), 2685–91. doi:10.1210/jcem.85.8.6755

Chu, J. Y. S., Cheng, C. Y. Y., Sekar, R., & Chow, B. K. C. (2013). Vagal afferent mediates the anorectic effect of peripheral secretin. *PloS One*, 8(5), e64859. doi:10.1371/journal.pone.0064859

Ciampolini, M., Lovell-Smith, D., Bianchi, R., de Pont, B., Sifone, M., van Weeren, M., . . . Pietrobelli, A. (2010). Sustained self-regulation of energy intake: Initial hunger improves insulin sensitivity. *Journal of Nutrition and Metabolism, 2010*. doi:10.1155/2010/286952

Ciampolini, M., Lovell-Smith, H. D., Kenealy, T., & Bianchi, R. (2013). Hunger can be taught: Hunger Recognition regulates eating and improves energy balance. *International Journal of General Medicine*, 6, 465–78. doi:10.2147/IJGM.S40655

Clegg, M. E., Pratt, M., Markey, O., Shafat, A., & Henry, C. J. K. (2012). Addition of different fats to a carbohydrate food: Impact on gastric emptying, glycaemic and satiety responses and comparison with in vitro digestion. *Food Research International*, 48(1), 91–97. doi:10.1016/j.foodres.2012.02.019

Dallman, M. F. (2010). Stress-induced obesity and the emotional nervous system. *Trends in Endocrinology and Metabolism: TEM*, 21(3), 159–65. doi:10.1016/j.tem.2009.10.004

De Graaf, C., Blom, W. A., Smeets, P. A., Stafleu, A., & Hendriks, H. F. (2004). Biomarkers of satiation and satiety. *American Journal of Clinical Nutrition*, 79(6), 946–61. Retrieved from http://ajcn.nutrition.org/content/79/6/946.full

Demos, K. E., Kelley, W. M., & Heatherton, T. F. (2011). Dietary restraint violations influence reward responses in nucleus accumbens and amygdala. *Journal of Cognitive Neuroscience*, 23(8), 1952–63. doi:10.1162/jocn.2010.21568

Dennis, E. A., Dengo, A. L., Comber, D. L., Flack, K. D., Savla, J., Davy, K. P., & Davy, B. M. (2010). Water consumption increases weight loss during a hypocaloric diet intervention in middle-aged and older adults. *Obesity* (Silver Spring, Md.), 18(2), 300–307. doi:10.1038/oby.2009.235

Drapeau, V., King, N., Hetherington, M., Doucet, E., Blundell, J., & Tremblay, A. (2007). Appetite sensations and satiety quotient: predictors of energy intake and weight loss. *Appetite*, 48(2), 159–66. doi:10.1016/j.appet.2006.08.002

Ebbeling, C. B., Feldman, H. A., Chomitz, V. R., Antonelli, T. A., Gortmaker, S. L., Osganian, S. K., & Ludwig, D. S. (2012). A randomized trial of sugar-sweetened beverages and adolescent body weight. *New England Journal of Medicine*, 367(15), 1407–16. doi:10.1056/NEJMoa1203388

Ebneter, D., Latner, J., Rosewall, J., & Chisholm, A. (2012). Impulsivity in restrained eaters : Emotional and external eating are associated with attentional and motor impulsivity. *Eat Weight Discord*. 2012; 17(1).

Engell, D., Kramer, M., Malafi, T., Salomon, M., & Lesher, L. (1996). Effects of effort and social modeling on drinking in humans. *Appetite*, 26(2), 129–38. doi:10.1006/appe.1996.0011

Evers, C., Marijn Stok, F., & de Ridder, D. T. D. (2010). Feeding your feelings: Emotion regulation strategies and emotional eating. *Personality & Social Psychology Bulletin*, 36(6), 792–804. doi:10.1177/0146167210371383

Figueiro, M. G., Plitnick, B., & Rea, M. S. (2012). Light modulates leptin and ghrelin in sleep-restricted adults. *International Journal of Endocrinology*, 2012, 530726. doi:10.1155/2012/530726

G Gregory Haff, M. J. L. (2003). Carbohydrate supplementation and resistance training. *Journal of Strength and Conditioning Research / National Strength & Conditioning Association*, 17(1), 187–96. doi:10.1519/1533-4287(2003)0172.0.CO;2

Gaetani, S., Fu, J., Cassano, T., Dipasquale, P., Romano, A., Righetti, L., . . . Piomelli, D. (2010). The fat-induced satiety factor oleoylethanolamide suppresses feeding through central release of oxytocin. *Journal of Neuroscience: The Official Journal of the Society for Neuroscience*, 30(24), 8096–101. doi:10.1523/JNEUROSCI.0036-10.2010

Gaetani, S., Oveisi, F., & Piomelli, D. (2003). Modulation of meal pattern in the rat by the anorexic lipid mediator oleoylethanolamide. *Neuropsychopharmacology: Official Publication of the American College of Neuropsychopharmacology*, 28(7), 1311–16. doi:10.1038/sj.npp.1300166

Geirsdottir, O. G., Arnarson, A., Ramel, A., Jonsson, P. V, & Thorsdottir, I. (2013). Dietary protein intake is associated with lean body mass in community-dwelling older adults. *Nutrition Research (New York, N.Y.)*, 33(8), 608–12. doi:10.1016/j.nutres.2013.05.014

Gibbons, C., Caudwell, P., Finlayson, G., Webb, D.-L., Hellström, P. M., Näslund, E., & Blundell, J. E. (2013). Comparison of postprandial profiles of ghrelin, active GLP-1, and total PYY to meals varying in fat and carbohydrate and their association with hunger and the phases of satiety. *Journal of Clinical Endocrinology and Metabolism*, 98(5), E847–55. doi:10.1210/jc.2012-3835

Ginsberg, H., Olefsky, J. M., Kimmerling, G., Crapo, P., & Reaven, G. M. (2013). Induction of hypertriglyceridemia by a low-fat diet. *The Journal of Clinical Endcrinology and Metabolism*, 42(4), 729–735

Gluck, M. E. (2006). Stress response and binge eating disorder. *Appetite*, 46(1), 26–30. doi:10.1016/j.appet.2005.05.004

Gluck, M. E., Geliebter, A., Hung, J., & Yahav, E. (2004). Cortisol, hunger, and desire to binge eat following a cold stress test in obese women with binge eating disorder. *Psychosomatic Medicine*, 66(6), 876–81. doi:10.1097/01.psy.0000143637.63508.47

Gopinath, B., Flood, V. M., Rochtchina, E., Baur, L. A., Louie, J. C. Y., Smith, W., & Mitchell, P. (2013). Carbohydrate nutrition and development of adiposity during adolescence. *Obesity* (Silver Spring, Md.), 21(9), 1884–90. doi:10.1002/oby.20405

Grandjean, A. C., Reimers, K. J., Bannick, K. E., & Haven, M. C. (2000). The effect of caffeinated, non-caffeinated, caloric and non-caloric beverages on hydration. *Journal of the American College of Nutrition*, 19(5), 591–600. http://www.ncbi.nlm.nih.gov/pubmed/11022872

Grandjean, A. C., Reimers, K. J., Haven, M. C., & Curtis, G. L. (2003). The effect on hydration of two diets, one with and one without plain water. *Journal of the American College of Nutrition*, 22(2), 165–73. Retrieved from http://www.ncbi.nlm.nih.gov/pubmed/12672713

Groesz, L. M., McCoy, S., Carl, J., Saslow, L., Stewart, J., Adler, N., . . . Epel, E. (2012). What is eating you? Stress and the drive to eat. *Appetite*, 58(2), 717–21. doi:10.1016/j.appet.2011.11.028

Gucht, D. Van, Soetens, B., Raes, F., & Griffith, J. W. (2014). The attitudes to chocolate questionnaire: psychometric properties and relationship with consumption, dieting, disinhibition and thought suppression. *Appetite*, (February). doi:10.1016/j.appet.2014.01.078

Haber, G. B., Heaton, K. W., Murphy, D., & Burroughs, L. F. (1977). Depletion and disruption of dietary fibre: Effects on satiety, plasma-glucose, and serum-insulin. *Lancet*, 2(8040), 679–82. http://www.ncbi.nlm.nih.gov/pubmed/71495

Hansen, H. S., & Diep, T. A. (2009). N-acylethanolamines, anandamide and food intake. *Biochemical Pharmacology*, 78(6), 553–60. doi:10.1016/j.bcp.2009.04.024

Harber, M. P., Konopka, A. R., Jemiolo, B., Trappe, S. W., Trappe, T. A., & Reidy, P. T. (2010). Muscle protein synthesis and gene expression during recovery from aerobic exercise in the fasted and fed states. *American Journal of Physiology. Regulatory, Integrative and Comparative Physiology*, 299(5), R1254–62. doi:10.1152/ajpregu.00348.2010

Hauner, H., Bechthold, A., Boeing, H., Brönstrup, A., Buyken, A., Leschik-Bonnet, E., . . . Wolfram, G. (2012). Evidence-based guideline of the German Nutrition Society: Carbohydrate intake and prevention of nutrition-related diseases. *Annals of Nutrition & Metabolism*, 60 Suppl 1, 1–58. doi:10.1159/000335326

Hawley, J. A., Burke, L. M., Phillips, S. M., & Spriet, L. L. (2011). Nutritional modulation of training-induced skeletal muscle adaptations. *Journal of Applied Physiology* (Bethesda, Md. : 1985), 110(3), 834–45. doi:10.1152/japplphysiol.00949.2010

He, W., Lam, T. K. T., Obici, S., & Rossetti, L. (2006). Molecular disruption of hypothalamic nutrient sensing induces obesity. *Nature Neuroscience*, 9(2), 227–33. doi:10.1038/nn1626

Heatherton, T. F., & Baumeister, R. F. (1991). Binge eating as escape from self-awareness. *Psychological Bulletin*, 110(1), 86–108. http://www.ncbi.nlm.nih.gov/pubmed/1891520

Herman, C. P., Fitzgerald, N. E., & Polivy, J. (2003). The influence of social norms on hunger ratings and eating. *Appetite*, 41(1), 15–20. doi:10.1016/S0195-6663(03)00027-8

Holt, S., Brand, J., Soveny, C., & Hansky, J. (1992). Relationship of satiety to postprandial glycaemic, insulin and cholecystokinin responses. *Appetite*, 18(2), 129–41. http://www.ncbi.nlm.nih.gov/pubmed/1610161

Hu, F. B., & Malik, V. S. (2010). Sugar-sweetened beverages and risk of obesity and type 2 diabetes: Epidemiologic evidence. *Physiology & Behavior*, 100(1), 47–54. doi:10.1016/j.physbeh.2010.01.036

Hu, J., La Vecchia, C., Augustin, L. S., Negri, E., de Groh, M., Morrison, H., & Mery, L. (2013). Glycemic index, glycemic load and cancer risk. *Annals of Oncology: Official Journal of the European Society for Medical Oncology / ESMO*, 24(1), 245–51. doi:10.1093/annonc/mds235

Hulston, C. J., Venables, M. C., Mann, C. H., Martin, C., Philp, A., Baar, K., & Jeukendrup, A. E. (2010). Training with low muscle glycogen enhances fat metabolism in well-trained cyclists. *Medicine and Science in Sports and Exercise*, 42(11), 2046–55. doi:10.1249/MSS.0b013e3181dd5070

Iwasaki, Y., & Yada, T. (2012). Vagal afferents sense meal-associated gastrointestinal and pancreatic hormones: Mechanism and physiological role. *Neuropeptides*, 46(6), 291–97. doi:10.1016/j.npep.2012.08.009

Kant, A. K. (2000). Consumption of energy-dense, nutrient-poor foods by adult Americans: Nutritional and health implications. The third National Health and Nutrition Examination Survey, 1988-1994. *American Journal of Clinical Nutrition*, 72(4), 929–36. http://www.ncbi.nlm.nih.gov/pubmed/11010933

Keim, N., Stern, J., & Havel, P. (1998). Relation between circulating leptin concentrations and appetite during a prolonged, moderate energy deficit in women. *American Journal of Clinical Nutrition*, 68(4), 794–801. http://ajcn.nutrition.org/content/68/4/794.abstract

Kim, C., & Pekrun, R. (2014). *Handbook of Research on Educational Communications and Technology*. (J. M. Spector, M. D. Merrill, J. Elen, & M. J. Bishop, Eds.) (pp. 65–75). New York: Springer New York. doi:10.1007/978-1-4614-3185-5

Koopman, K. E., Booij, J., Fliers, E., Serlie, M. J., & la Fleur, S. E. (2013). Diet-induced changes in the Lean Brain: Hypercaloric high-fat-high-sugar snacking decreases serotonin transporters in the human hypothalamic region. *Molecular Metabolism*, 2(4), 417–22. doi:10.1016/j.molmet.2013.07.006

Kulovitz, M. G., Kravitz, L. R., Mermier, C., Gibson, A. L., Conn, C. A, Kolkmeyer, D., & Kerksick, C. M. (2013). Potential role of meal frequency as a strategy for weight loss and health in overweight or obese adults. *Nutrition* (Burbank, Los Angeles County, Calif.), 1–7. doi:10.1016/j.nut.2013.08.009

Lam, T. K. T., Schwartz, G. J., & Rossetti, L. (2005). Hypothalamic sensing of fatty acids. *Nature Neuroscience*, 8(5), 579–84. doi:10.1038/nn1456

Lambert, E. V., Goedecke, J. H., Zyle, C., Murphy, K., Hawley, J. A., Dennis, S. C., & Noakes, T. D. (2001). High-fat diet versus habitual diet prior to carbohydrate loading: Effects of exercise metabolism and cycling performance. *International Journal of Sport Nutrition and Exercise Metabolism*, 11(2), 209–25. http://www.ncbi.nlm.nih.gov/pubmed/11402254

Lappalainen, R., Mennen, L., van Weert, L., & Mykkänen, H. (1993). Drinking water with a meal: A simple method of coping with feelings of hunger, satiety and desire to eat. *European Journal of Clinical Nutrition*, 47(11), 815–9. http://www.ncbi.nlm.nih.gov/pubmed/8287852

Ledikwe, J. H., Blanck, H. M., Kettel Khan, L., Serdula, M. K., Seymour, J. D., Tohill, B. C., & Rolls, B. J. (2006). Dietary energy density is associated with energy intake and weight status in US adults. *American Journal of Clinical Nutrition*, 83(6), 1362–68. http://www.ncbi.nlm.nih.gov/pubmed/16762948

Leidy, H. J., Armstrong, C. L. H., Tang, M., Mattes, R. D., & Campbell, W. W. (2010). The influence of higher protein intake and greater eating frequency on appetite control in overweight and obese men. *Obesity* (Silver Spring, Md.), 18(9), 1725–32. doi:10.1038/oby.2010.45

Leidy, H. J., Carnell, N. S., Mattes, R. D., & Campbell, W. W. (2007). Higher protein intake preserves lean mass and satiety with weight loss in pre-obese and obese women. *Obesity* (Silver Spring, Md.), 15(2), 421–29. doi:10.1038/oby.2007.531

Leidy, H. J., Mattes, R. D., & Campbell, W. W. (2007). Effects of acute and chronic protein intake on metabolism, appetite, and ghrelin during weight loss. *Obesity* (Silver Spring, Md.), 15(5), 1215–25. doi:10.1038/oby.2007.143

Leidy, H. J., Tang, M., Armstrong, C. L. H., Martin, C. B., & Campbell, W. W. (2009). The effects of consuming frequent, higher protein meals on appetite and satiety during weight loss in overweight/obese men. *Obesity*, 19(4), 818–24. doi:10.1038/oby.2010.203

Lejeune, M. P., Westerterp, K. R., Adam, T. C., Luscombe-Marsh, N. D., & Westerterp-Plantenga, M. S. (2006). Ghrelin and glucagon-like peptide 1 concentrations, 24-h satiety, and energy and substrate metabolism during a high-protein diet and measured in a respiration chamber. *American Journal of Clinical Nutrition*, 83(1), 89–94. http://ajcn.nutrition.org/content/83/1/89.full

Lennerz, B. S., Alsop, D. C., Holsen, L. M., Stern, E., Rojas, R., Ebbeling, C. B., . . . Ludwig, D. S. (2013). Effects of dietary glycemic index on brain regions related to reward and craving in men. *The American Journal of Clinical Nutrition*, 98(3), 641–47. doi:10.3945/ajcn.113.064113

Lissner, L., Levitsky, D., Strupp, B., Kalkwarf, H., & Roe, D. (1987). Dietary fat and the regulation of energy intake in human subjects. *American Journal of Clinical Nutrition*, 46(6), 886–92. http://ajcn.nutrition.org/content/46/6/886.abstract

Little, T. J., & Feinle-Bisset, C. (2010). Oral and gastrointestinal sensing of dietary fat and appetite regulation in humans: Modification by diet and obesity. *Frontiers in Neuroscience*, 4, 178. doi:10.3389/fnins.2010.00178

Liu, S., Manson, J. E., Buring, J. E., Stampfer, M. J., Willett, W. C., & Ridker, P. M. (2002). Relation between a diet with a high glycemic load and plasma concentrations of high-sensitivity C-reactive protein in middle-aged women. *American Journal of Clinical Nutrition*, 75(3), 492–498. http://ajcn.nutrition.org/content/75/3/492.full

Loenneke, J. P., Wilson, J. M., Manninen, A. H., Wray, M. E., Barnes, J. T., & Pujol, T. J. (2012). Quality protein intake is inversely related with abdominal fat. *Nutrition & Metabolism*, 9(1), 5. doi:10.1186/1743-7075-9-5

Lovell-Smith, D., Kenealy, T., & Buetow, S. (2010). Eating when empty is good for your health. *Medical Hypotheses*, 75(2), 172–78. doi:10.1016/j.mehy.2010.02.013

Ludwig, D. S. (2000). Dietary Glycemic Index and Obesity. *Journal Nutrition.*, 130(2), p.280S—283S. http://jn.nutrition.org/content/130/2/280S.full

Ludwig, D. S., Majzoub, J. A., Al-Zahrani, A., Dallal, G. E., Blanco, I., & Roberts, S. B. (1999). High glycemic index foods, overeating, and obesity. *Pediatrics*, 103(3), p.E26. doi:10.1542/peds.103.3.e26

Madden, C. E. L., Leong, S. L., Gray, A., & Horwath, C. C. (2012). Eating in response to hunger and satiety signals is related to BMI in a nationwide sample of 1601 mid-age New Zealand women. *Public Health Nutrition*, 15(12), 2272–9. doi:10.1017/S1368980012000882

Maffeis, C., Bonadonna, R., Maschio, M., Aiello, G., Tommasi, M., Marigliano, M., … Morandi, A. (2013). Metabolic and hormonal consequences of two different meals after a moderate intensity exercise bout in obese prepubertal children. *European Journal of Clinical Nutrition*, 67(7), 725–31. doi:10.1038/ejcn.2013.86

Malik, V. S., & Hu, F. B. (2012). Sweeteners and risk of bbesity and type 2 diabetes: The Role of sugar-sweetened beverages. *Current Diabetes Reports.* doi:10.1007/s11892-012-0259-6

Markwald, R. R., Melanson, E. L., Smith, M. R., Higgins, J., Perreault, L., Eckel, R. H., & Wright, K. P. (2013). Impact of insufficient sleep on total daily energy expenditure, food intake, and weight gain. *Proceedings of the National Academy of Sciences of the United States of America*, 110(14), 5695–700. doi:10.1073/pnas.1216951110

Marmonier, C., Chapelot, D., Fantino, M., & Louis-Sylvestre, J. (2002). Snacks consumed in a nonhungry state have poor satiating efficiency: Influence of snack composition on substrate utilization. *American Journal of Clinical Nutrition*, 76(3) p.518–528.

Martens, E. A., Lemmens, S. G., & Westerterp-Plantenga, M. S. (2013). Protein leverage affects energy intake of high-protein diets in humans. *American Journal of Clinical Nutrition*, 97(1), 86–93. doi:10.3945/ajcn.112.046540

McClain, A. D., Otten, J. J., Hekler, E. B., & Gardner, C. D. (2013). Adherence to a low-fat vs. low-carbohydrate diet differs by insulin resistance status. *Diabetes, Obesity & Metabolism*, 15(1), 87–90. doi:10.1111/j.1463-1326.2012.01668.x

McIver, C. M., Wycherley, T. P., & Clifton, P. M. (2012). MTOR signaling and ubiquitin-proteosome gene expression in the preservation of fat free mass following high protein, calorie restricted weight loss. *Nutrition & Metabolism*, 9(1), 83. doi:10.1186/1743-7075-9-83

McKiernan, F., Houchins, J. A., & Mattes, R. D. (2008). Relationships between human thirst, hunger, drinking, and feeding. *Physiology & Behavior*, 94(5), 700–708. doi:10.1016/j.physbeh.2008.04.007

McManus, K., Antinoro, L., & Sacks, F. (2001). A randomized controlled trial of a moderate-fat, low-energy diet compared with a low fat, low-energy diet for weight loss in overweight adults. *International Journal of Obesity and Related Metabolic Disorders : Journal of the International Association for the Study of Obesity*, 25(10), 1503–11. doi:10.1038/sj.ijo.0801796

Melby, C. L., Osterberg, K. L., Resch, A., Davy, B., Johnson, S., & Davy, K. (2002). Effect of carbohydrate ingestion during exercise on post-exercise substrate oxidation and energy intake. *International Journal of Sport Nutrition and Exercise Metabolism*, 12(3), 294–309. http://www.ncbi.nlm.nih.gov/pubmed/12432174

Monteiro, C. A., Levy, R. B., Claro, R. M., de Castro, I. R. R., & Cannon, G. (2011). Increasing consumption of ultra-processed foods and likely impact on human health: Evidence from Brazil. *Public Health Nutrition*, 14(1), 5–13. doi:10.1017/S1368980010003241

Moubarac, J.-C., Martins, A. P. B., Claro, R. M., Levy, R. B., Cannon, G., & Monteiro, C. A. (2013). Consumption of ultra-processed foods and likely impact on human health: Evidence from Canada. *Public Health Nutrition*, 16(12), 2240–48. doi:10.1017/S1368980012005009

Munsters, M. J. M., & Saris, W. H. M. (2012). Effects of meal frequency on metabolic profiles and substrate partitioning in lean healthy males. *PLoS ONE*, 7(6), e38632. doi:10.1371/journal.pone.0038632

Murray, M., & Vickers, Z. (2009). Consumer views of hunger and fullness: A qualitative approach. *Appetite*, 53(2), 174–82. doi:10.1016/j.appet.2009.06.003

Näslund, E., Barkeling, B., King, N., Gutniak, M., Blundell, J. E., Holst, J. J., . . . Hellström, P. M. (1999). Energy intake and appetite are suppressed by glucagon-like peptide-1 (GLP-1) in obese men. *International Journal of Obesity and Related Metabolic Disorders: Journal of the International Association for the Study of Obesity*, 23(3), 304–11. http://www.ncbi.nlm.nih.gov/pubmed/10193877

Nevanperä, N., Lappalainen, R., Kuosma, E., Hopsu, L., Uitti, J., & Laitinen, J. (2013). Psychological flexibility, occupational burnout and eating behavior among working women. *Open Journal of Preventive Medicine*, 03(04), 355–61. doi:10.4236/ojpm.2013.34048

Ohkawara, K., Cornier, M.-A., Kohrt, W. M., & Melanson, E. L. (2013). Effects of increased meal frequency on fat oxidation and perceived hunger. *Obesity* (Silver Spring, Md.), 21(2), 336–43. doi:10.1002/oby.20032

Pan, A., & Hu, F. B. (2011). Effects of carbohydrates on satiety: Differences between liquid and solid food. *Current Opinion in Clinical Nutrition and Metabolic Care*, 14(4), 385–90. doi:10.1097/MCO.0b013e328346df36

Pan, A., Malik, V. S., Hao, T., Willett, W. C., Mozaffarian, D., & Hu, F. B. (2013). Changes in water and beverage intake and long-term weight changes: Results from three prospective cohort studies. *International Journal of Obesity (2005)*, 37(10), 1378–85. doi:10.1038/ijo.2012.225

Pasman, W. J., van Erk, M. J., Klöpping, W. A. A., Pellis, L., Wopereis, S., Bijlsma, S., ... Kardinaal, A. F. M. (2013). Nutrigenomics approach elucidates health-promoting effects of high vegetable intake in lean and obese men. *Genes & Nutrition*, 8(5), 507–21. doi:10.1007/s12263-013-0343-9

Pelkman, C. L., Fishell, V. K., Maddox, D. H., Pearson, T. A., Mauger, D. T., & Kris-Etherton, P. M. (2004). Effects of moderate-fat (from monounsaturated fat) and low-fat weight-loss diets on the serum lipid profile in overweight and obese men and women. *American Journal of Clinical Nutrition*, 79(2), 204–12. http://ajcn.nutrition.org/content/79/2/204.full

Piomelli, D. (2013). A fatty gut feeling. *Trends in Endocrinology and Metabolism: TEM*, 24(7), 332–41. doi:10.1016/j.tem.2013.03.001

Pittas, A. G., Hariharan, R., Stark, P. C., Hajduk, C. L., Greenberg, A. S., & Roberts, S. B. (2005). Interstitial glucose level is a significant predictor of energy intake in free-living women with healthy body weight. *Journal Nutrition.*, 135(5), 1070–74. http://jn.nutrition.org/content/135/5/1070.full

Popkin, B. M., Barclay, D. V, & Nielsen, S. J. (2005). Water and food consumption patterns of U.S. adults from 1999 to 2001. *Obesity Research*, 13(12), 2146–52. doi:10.1038/oby.2005.266

Popkin, B. M., & Duffey, K. J. (2010). Does hunger and satiety drive eating anymore? Increasing eating occasions and decreasing time between eating occasions in the United States. *American Journal of Clinical Nutrition*, 91(5), 1342–1347.

Romano, A., Cassano, T., Tempesta, B., Cianci, S., Dipasquale, P., Coccurello, R., . . . Gaetani, S. (2013). The satiety signal oleoylethanolamide stimulates oxytocin neurosecretion from rat hypothalamic neurons. *Peptides*, 49, 21–26. doi:10.1016/j.peptides.2013.08.006

Rosenbaum, M., & Leibel, R. L. (2010). Adaptive thermogenesis in humans. *International Journal of Obesity (2005)*, 34 Suppl 1, S47–55. doi:10.1038/ijo.2010.184

Rutters, F., Nieuwenhuizen, A. G., Lemmens, S. G. T., Born, J. M., & Westerterp-Plantenga, M. S. (2009). Acute stress-related changes in eating in the absence of hunger. *Obesity* (Silver Spring, Md.), 17(1), 72–77. doi:10.1038/oby.2008.493

Ryan, A. T., Feinle-Bisset, C., Kallas, A., Wishart, J. M., Clifton, P. M., Horowitz, M., & Luscombe-Marsh, N. D. (2012). Intraduodenal protein modulates antropyloroduodenal motility, hormone release, glycemia, appetite, and energy intake in lean men. *American Journal of Clinical Nutrition*, 96(3), 474–82. doi:10.3945/ajcn.112.038133

Ryan, A. T., Luscombe-Marsh, N. D., Saies, A. A., Little, T. J., Standfield, S., Horowitz, M., & Feinle-Bisset, C. (2013). Effects of intraduodenal lipid and protein on gut motility and hormone release, glycemia, appetite, and energy intake in lean men. *The American Journal of Clinical Nutrition*, 98(2), 300–311. doi:10.3945/ajcn.113.061333

Sarro-Ramírez, A., Sánchez-López, D., Tejeda-Padrón, A., Frías, C., Zaldívar-Rae, J., & Murillo-Rodríguez, E. (2013). Brain molecules and appetite: The case of oleoylethanolamide. *Central Nervous System Agents in Medicinal Chemistry*, 13(1), 88–91. http://www.ncbi.nlm.nih.gov/pubmed/23464987

Savage, J., Marini, M., & Birch, L. (2008). Dietary energy density predicts women's weight change over 6 y 1–3. *The American Journal of Clinical Nutrition*, 88(3), p.677-684.

Schwartz, G. J., Fu, J., Astarita, G., Li, X., Gaetani, S., Campolongo, P., . . . Piomelli, D. (2008). The lipid messenger OEA links dietary fat intake to satiety. *Cell Metabolism*, 8(4), 281–88. doi:10.1016/j.cmet.2008.08.005

Schwarzfuchs, D., Golan, R., & Shai, I. (2012). Four-year follow-up after two-year dietary interventions. *The New England Journal of Medicine*, 367(14), 1373–4. doi:10.1056/NEJMc1204792

Shai, I., Schwarzfuchs, D., Henkin, Y., Shahar, D. R., Witkow, S., Greenberg, I., ... Stampfer, M. J. (2008). Weight loss with a low-carbohydrate, Mediterranean, or low-fat diet. *The New England Journal of Medicine*, 359(3), 229–41. doi:10.1056/NEJMoa0708681

Shughrue, P. J., Lane, M. V, & Merchenthaler, I. (1996). Glucagon-like peptide-1 receptor (GLP1-R) mRNA in the rat hypothalamus. *Endocrinology*, 137(11), 5159–62. doi:10.1210/endo.137.11.8895391

Sieri, S., Brighenti, F., Agnoli, C., Grioni, S., Masala, G., Bendinelli, B., . . . Krogh, V. (2013). Dietary glycemic load and glycemic index and risk of cerebrovascular disease in the EPICOR cohort. *PloS One*, 8(5), e62625. doi:10.1371/journal.pone.0062625

Sluijs, I., van der Schouw, Y. T., van der A, D. L., Spijkerman, A. M., Hu, F. B., Grobbee, D. E., & Beulens, J. W. (2010). Carbohydrate quantity and quality and risk of type 2 diabetes in the European Prospective Investigation into Cancer and Nutrition-Netherlands (EPIC-NL) study. *The American Journal of Clinical Nutrition*, 92(4), 905–11. doi:10.3945/ajcn.2010.29620

Smith, C. F., Williamson, D. A, Bray, G. A, & Ryan, D. H. (1999). Flexible vs. Rigid dieting strategies: relationship with adverse behavioral outcomes. *Appetite*, 32(3), 295–305. doi:10.1006/appe.1998.0204

Solomon, T. P. J., Chambers, E. S., Jeukendrup, A. E., Toogood, A. A, & Blannin, A. K. (2008). The effect of feeding frequency on insulin and ghrelin responses in human subjects. *The British Journal of Nutrition*, 100(4), 810–19. doi:10.1017/S000711450896757X

Song, S. W., Bae, Y. J., & Lee, D. T. (2010). Effects of caloric restriction with varying energy density and aerobic exercise on weight change and satiety in young female adults. *Nutrition Research and Practice*, 4(5), 414–20. doi:10.4162/nrp.2010.4.5.414

Spaeth, A. M., Dinges, D. F., & Goel, N. (2013). Effects of experimental sleep restriction on weight gain, caloric intake, and meal timing in healthy adults. *Sleep*, 36(7), 981–90. doi:10.5665/sleep.2792

Spiegel, K. (2004). Brief communication: Sleep curtailment in healthy young men is associated with decreased leptin levels, elevated ghrelin levels, and increased hunger and appetite. *Annals of Internal Medicine*, 141(11), 846. doi:10.7326/0003-4819-141-11-200412070-00008

Spiegel, K., Leproult, R., L'hermite-Balériaux, M., Copinschi, G., Penev, P. D., & Van Cauter, E. (2004). Leptin levels are dependent on sleep duration: Relationships with sympathovagal balance, carbohydrate regulation, cortisol, and thyrotropin. *Journal of Clinical Endocrinology and Metabolism*, 89(11), 5762–71. doi:10.1210/jc.2004-1003

St.-Onge, M.-P., Roberts, A. L., Chen, J., Kelleman, M., O'Keeffe, M., RoyChoudhury, A., & Jones, P. J. H. (2011). Short sleep duration increases energy intakes but does not change energy expenditure in normal-weight individuals. *The American Journal of Clinical Nutrition*, 94(2), 410–16. doi:10.3945/ajcn.111.013904

Tellez, L. A., Medina, S., Han, W., Ferreira, J. G., Licona-Limón, P., Ren, X., . . . de Araujo, I. E. (2013). A gut lipid messenger links excess dietary fat to dopamine deficiency. *Science* (New York, N.Y.), *341*(6147), 800–802. doi:10.1126/science.1239275

Tomiyama, A. J., Mann, T., Vinas, D., Hunger, J. M., Dejager, J., & Taylor, S. E. (2010). Low calorie dieting increases cortisol. *Psychosomatic Medicine*, 72(4), 357–64. doi:10.1097/PSY.0b013e3181d9523c

Tomiyama, A. J., Schamarek, I., Lustig, R. H., Kirschbaum, C., Puterman, E., Havel, P. J., & Epel, E. S. (2012). Leptin concentrations in response to acute stress predict subsequent intake of comfort foods. *Physiology & Behavior*, 107(1), 34–9. doi:10.1016/j.physbeh.2012.04.021

Toshinai, K., Mondal, M. S., Shimbara, T., Yamaguchi, H., Date, Y., Kangawa, K., & Nakazato, M. (2007). Ghrelin stimulates growth hormone secretion and food intake in aged rats. *Mechanisms of Ageing and Development*, 128(2), 182–86. doi:10.1016/j.mad.2006.10.001

Tsintzas, K., & Williams, C. (1998). Human muscle glycogen metabolism during exercise: Effect of carbohydrate supplementation. *Sports Medicine (Auckland, N.Z.)*, 25(1), 7–23. http://www.ncbi.nlm.nih.gov/pubmed/9458524

Volkow, N. D., Wang, G.-J., & Baler, R. D. (2011). Reward, dopamine and the control of food intake: Implications for obesity. *Trends in Cognitive Sciences*, 15(1), 37–46. doi:10.1016/j.tics.2010.11.001

Wagner, D. D., Boswell, R. G., Kelley, W. M., & Heatherton, T. F. (2012). Inducing negative affect increases the reward value of appetizing foods in dieters. *Journal of Cognitive Neuroscience*, 24(7), 1625–33. doi:10.1162/jocn_a_00238

Walsh, C. O., Ebbeling, C. B., Swain, J. F., Markowitz, R. L., Feldman, H. A., & Ludwig, D. S. (2013). Effects of diet composition on postprandial energy availability during weight loss maintenance. *PloS One*, 8(3), e58172. doi:10.1371/journal.pone.0058172

Williams, R. A., Roe, L. S., & Rolls, B. J. (2013). Comparison of three methods to reduce energy density. Effects on daily energy intake. *Appetite*, 66, 75–83. doi:10.1016/j.appet.2013.03.004

ACKNOWLEDGMENTS

Without the support and encouragement of my husband, Roland Fisher, this book (and many other things in my life) would not have been possible. Thank you to Brandice Lardner and Kara Beutel for their contributions, creativity and passion for coaching; you make me a better coach daily. Thank you Janna Stam and Diane Snyder for your skilled eyes in revising and helping me improve the clarity of my writing. My agent Linda Konner has been an invaluable team member, and I appreciate her expertise and guidance in all my writing projects. Last, thank you Marissa, William and all the delightful people at Page Street for your commitment to excellence and a shared ambition to produce the finest books possible. It has been an absolute pleasure, from start to finish, to partner with Page Street.

ABOUT THE AUTHOR

Georgie Fear is a registered dietitian and professional nutrition coach. A co-founder of One By One Nutrition, Georgie uses her habit-based change approach to help clients around the world achieve lifelong weight-loss success without restrictive dieting. In addition to her interpersonal coaching skill, she is well known for combining her scientific expertise with loving, kind and levelheaded support through her writing. A native of New Jersey and Colorado, Georgie and her husband, Roland Fisher, now live in beautiful Vancouver, British Columbia. Stop by onebyonenutrition.com for more of Georgie's work.

INDEX